STRANDS OF MY LOVER'S HAIR

GW00976160

By Matthew Woods

best wishes

Matthew Woods

"One million people commit suicide every year."
The World Health Organisation

Published by:
Chipmunkapublishing
PO Box 6872
Brentwood
Essex
CM13 1ZT
United Kingdom

http://www.chipmunkapublishing.com

PART ONE: The Meteor Seed

Chapter. 1 Ivory Towers

Misty desire arose as fireflies beat out that life is time's fool. Their chaotic fools' life of a day burning brightly to attract a mate. But is ours so different? *Love only made one believe in what won't happen and proved nothing to be true© Oscar Wilde.* By merely elapsing time makes nonsense of all life's conscious planning and scheming. Love is too impractical. Only where it is possible to ignore individuals and consider only large numbers and the law of averages, is any kind of accurate foresight possible and with the passage of time the variables tend to increase in number and change their character. One cannot change what one regrets from our ivory towers, so pert and glistening, bitter rust gleaming bright. They believed that strength was hidden in decorum not freedom. Indeed the only constant was that of time in the sparking and winking of cameras, which they greedily consumed as life diminished into possessions. A feature of their journey was only one real cousin of presumption-the appropriate. To do as one ought. Human behavior faced with time decided in the logical realms of the cushioned, sickening reliance upon sanity and washed up as its victims. Perhaps the only way to appreciate genuine time is to have the tumultuous tortured imagination to link the void of the world to your psyche. They would appreciate care but not the true meaning of sentiment. They were stuck in their ivory tower.

This was not lost on Michael. The pilot of our story was a hero-at-zero. He wondered if his decision of the bitter end, which he only had the inkling of at the moment, was that part of him which adhered to reputation. It was the bitter rust, gleaming bright; a split after four years due to his arrogance. The birds on the wing told of the love he was leaving that it was a crime against nature to leave the honesty and beauty, which had given him so much loyalty. He did not and would never know that it had also given him a child. They told him to pick her up in his arms and hold her, kiss her and comfort her. Tears welled up in his eyes as the stark reality of his decision turned his emotions to the definition of his life. A dangerous mysterious existence that left only himself to rely upon, implacable and dynamic. He got up, shaved and left the tower knowing he would only return to say his goodbyes.

A faith in love's dream, heaven and earth, God, queen and country, as simple as a woolly, changed only when placed in certain circumstances. A white lie, cloud grey was something only a lover will have noticed in the skies where only lovers die. Flibbertigibbet undresses each night in her tower and resumes the V-neck jumper in the morning. These insistent little habits brought ones motives into play; she papered the real tracts of her tears to bear on the woolly wedlock of spirit and mind. The view from the Martello tower unveiled the unholy patchwork of the Essex fields and the sea, the woolen clouds; the ley lines of a county at the speed of sound; strange forms of excitement mixed with fear, converse loyalties and reverie arose from the vertigo heights.

Michael pushed out his remorse and climbed into his MG. The familiar raucous of the engine freed him from the Cleopatra grip and as he sped along the sun and wind which conveyed the pushing out of the feelings he had achieved. As he entered Waterbeach gates he did up his buttons with his free hand and quite forgot the pain he had experienced. What would she miss anyway? He thought. Those who were alone were left outside- the last thing he needed was reassurance from a woman stuck in her ivory tower. He couldn't stand the possessiveness. He would only be hovering over the remains of the chase. The whole experience of love had been a chase and perhaps that was all he had left. He had fallen in love with the girl but now he feared the effects of his crippling rejection. He could dance with her until he didn't exist and it still wouldn't make any difference.

"The floundering returns then" said Peter. Michael had landed badly yesterday and Peter was not going to let him forget it. They had both trained on chipmunks and these were forgiving aircrafts but they tended to be prone to crosswind on landing, being light but manoeuvrable.

"What about you then, swooping around like sheets of rain?" Their rivalry was just in fun and constantly argued. They were however impatient to turn their hands at the dogfights, which were the backbone of 56th squadron, and they had a tendency to turn a glassy blind eye to the rulebook if they didn't get their way. Beneath the late 40's sun they had begun their training. They had enjoyed a fair few hours flight but mostly they practiced unwieldy processional flying which was a laborious formality in the empty skies above Essex. It was boring.

    This was probably what the briefing was about, attack formation and they had had enough of the techniques of locating neighbouring planes and the distances to keep. The senior members in the squadron passed on theory and practice and the differences between, on social time, so as Peter thought, they learnt more from the shindigs afterwards. Michael however had his mind on other things and as he stared at this morning's business, he drifted off. They called him crow because of his nose pursed like a beak under his pale, grey piercing eyes. Michael closed his eyes.

    There was a tree, which stood upon a grassy knoll. All logic had his eye on the tree, for its majestic beauty overwhelmed him and he wanted to turn it into a piano. Its roots were a massed and tangled pathway through which life was fingered by all the children who played around it. They captured its fruits for even the fruit that doesn't want to be eaten will still fall off the tree. All logic swung its forefinger over his palm and swung the axe countless, fruitless times over the years but he only touched it as had a stone to skim on the waters of despair. Its hand needed a lily-white hand to close over his, because this hand would protect him, so he felt self-respect no more, and through this the both of them could fell the tree. The suffering flowed like water over Excalibur and out of the tree a hand emerged; the hand began to play on the axe. The void flew from cover as the hand began to speak of love and everything they knew. But the lily-white hand was a hand that protected, protected from the mouth which spoke desire, stranger than kindness. The speaking hand continued to wither winter's cold and melody beckoned, carelessly close.

The tune asked where time had gone as they swung the axe, but the tree just loomed like fate to say I am coming back to you, from where we started, from where they came from; a dream and truth to the way back home. The hand was a ghost seeping from the form of the tree and disappearing into the sky, beauty, impossible to define, impossible to believe, to endure beneath its chords. The feeling of flying gracefully above the clouds engulfed him and such the composer knew was no longer written. However there was a vortex with a beautiful melody drawing him to swoop lower and lower towards it; in his path it was deceptions twin, inspirations kin, improvisations sin and I let them in. It criticized my torment through my disguise. The wind did howl among the deep brown boughs and the wind did peel majors and minors from its kiss. The song was the punishment of my present self. He wrote the only words he could on the bough "I love you" and the melancholy stopped, the tune that was too beautiful to endure, too beautiful to believe played no more. Dull to the crying thigh, the tree lurched and drew its roots from the ground. He focused himself. The tree he had spent 20 years chopping down suddenly toppled and like silence fell on his back.

Michael started with a jolt. Flight commander Brodie was staring at him and had obviously asked him a question. "Well" he asked expectantly. "What is it with you, sergeant pilot Warrick, woman trouble?" Anyway it was his life he was living now. He would tell her, sometime. His was of freedom and self-expression, speed and thrill. It had been a good year for the roses. They were soon out on the tarmac. The meteors stood proud and gleaming on the runway and the cloud hung low. They were to practice a few manoeuvres one of which was the *rhubarb* that was to hide among the layer of cloud and quickly dive from cover. The main business of the day was in following drogues and the meteors would unleash their guns today.

Quickly he clipped his straps and pressed the starter button; the engine engulfed the serenity like thunder, and he was winding his trimming wheel as he went booming past the grass verge- with a rending the nose was airborne. The strange sensation of a tight chest and elation followed the take off. Indeed contradictions of fear and elation lay under the surface like sinews in a naked body but always decently covered with understatement. Michael saw control of fear as the best instrument in his cockpit. Two meteors closed fast and one opened up the throttle for its flanks to dart past. It was Peter. They ascended in formation. Acrobatics were frowned upon and no pilot was too eager to cross Brodie's wrath but each pilot had to do the *gamecock* at least once a month, the most dangerous of maneuvers with the speed and power of a jet engine. It was to pull up in a loop, flick roll into a spin at the top and hopefully pull out and complete the loop.

In dogfights every pilot knew that the chap who got in close could bring them down. Over the mike came the ominous- *angel 5, line astern, line astern!* And the planes would turn around in the cockpit and present his belly for a sitting shot then be left up to their own initiative to dive out of trouble. Coming back from a sweep he noticed his thoughts were flashing across his mind very quickly. He rose and climbed to the cloud ceiling and went after the drogues. He darted down out of the sun on each side of a target plane and breaking sharply forwards and underneath. After that came the rattling of the machine guns as each drogue was systematically riddled with bullets.

Days of dogfight practice came and went interspersed with convoy missions and other routine patrols. Thankfully the meteors all avoided all sign of dead stick except for one crisp morning when he had to make an emergency landing. The picture of him standing by his downed plane was proudly put in the clubhouse with the rest of the near fatalities. On that day he confronted his feelings and spoke to the woman he had loved for so long. "There's something very self satisfied about you which you do not learn from" she began after he had met her in the local.

"The trouble is I talk as if I care but as you say we're worlds apart now".

"Though the same environment of compassion, confidence, happiness and sorrow surely", she said. So used to pitting reserve against the odds all he could say was "no" and with that they silently drank their drinks. Parting never was such sweet sorrow. It may have been the heady lunacy of her ivory tower, but she never told him she was pregnant.

Michael went off to watch a Doris Day film. Pretentious and false she may be but certainly reliable. Let it snow, let it snow, let it snow! Michael proved to be reliable in the squadron and it was an exciting period for aviation. The Americans were developing Nazi ideas on the swept back wing, engine technology was progressing rapidly and the civil airliners were reaching economical readiness. The madness in her heart touched Michael whose romantic ideals continued. She stared down from her tower and fingered a shell she had collected from the beach.

The shell and she
Indivisible as one
Pale and smooth inside
Its faithful fragility
She caresses as though it were he
She caresses the lip
She caresses her soul to begin

She and the shell

The shell and she
Caressed by the warmth of the sea
As the sea caresses the ship
As a weaver her spell to spin
Hush and you will see
Poseidon's grip
Her as a flaxen figurine
She and the shell

The shell and she
Held in her fragile majesty
Pulls the sailor from the ship
Emerging from the water's Breen
A spell to caste momentarily
And land us here forsaken
As Venus from her shell emerges
She and the shell

The meteor always had something of a reputation for being slow, large and unwieldy- but it was the plane of choice in the right hands. It had proved the ascendance of Whittle's jet engine. Michael remained part of the elite squadron based at Waterbeach, which combined the strength of American and English pilots. He had a chance to fly the Sabre. He was living in luxury at the officer's mess- if one could stand the bilge of formality, stewards would rush around to see to your requisites. The bachelor's life was well catered for. Everyone called you sir and the plush lifestyle was not too far away from how life should be. Which brings us to the formation flypast over London on Coronation day 1952. So all that practice wasn't useless then, he thought.

His plane soared gracefully with throttle idling. Over the quiet houses he flew and the boxes below him looked like secluded orange groves to a bee. He came within sight of the Thames in close formation and the procession of the queen's coronation carriage was a glorified trail of ants. He felt like he was a page of history and with a roar of the engines he passed over the houses of Parliament where he knew his family were watching. She was more than just some name on a pub sign. Their ivory towers were ruled by the pomp of moderation like a good English beer.

He was returning to his base passing over the area he lived to barnstorm his father's house when he swept over the forest. As he did so a strange feeling welled up in him. A tree seemed to stand out, grew as if he were being strangled by the forests intertwining leaves. A vortex flew towards him. It swallowed up his craft in a pinnacle of light. He and his plane were no longer there. As he disappeared there was a rare occurrence. Something that only happened in destiny. Ned was born, breaking the quiet with a scream.

From former to now
From land to sea
And fondly the soul we
The home of our tower

Wantonly fermenting
The brew of my form
Now the ear has frequented
The space between land and sea
A tumultuous coven of equinox
A stray child is born
From after to then
From land to sea
Lushly the breath shelters
The home of our tower
Fervently creating
The blush of your warmth
Now the ear has frequented
The space between land and sea
A tumultuous coven of equinox
A stray child is born

As Flibbertigibbet stands forlorn in her ivory tower, I woke up with pride not braveness. Can the truth be told by a throttle? There is only one difference between a woman and a bottle; the hand rests well in both, but a woman has more cruel. A crawling woman and a bottle are both heaven and destruction. You said you preferred the loneliness of your tower. They've pulled down the café where we used to meet. The bombed out buildings were my feelings of rejection, firmly compounded by loyalty in perfection, for yet another apocalyptic air display. As deliquesce aircraft did acrobatics you insisted upon standing with your Rubicon, lost in remembrance of you bare, all occurring the same time somewhere, overcome by the darkening air. She asked if her crutch was like Egypt- for when you leave like this, it's quite timeless; like fragments of a roller coaster ride, seamless. Her kisses mocked her troubles, endearing, concise and gullible, and we carried on in this trinity tower. A beauty I'd always miss with these eyes before.

As Flibbertigibbet stands forlorn in her ivory tower, the man who was paint on the ceiling talked of staying and left; I talked of leaving but stayed; on the fringe of a circle, mottled from most but from the inside, on a fringe of light he felt falling from the clouds, on a fringe of the sights and sounds emanating from the view from the tower, something was becoming hot on the wire. He was seeing the clement, captivating nurture of her face, her fringe delicately softened. I can't answer your tragical questions through the mists and visions of time. Show her that her ivory tower was my secret love for her.

Chapter 2 A Blood Perihelion

Holding forever the dead moon, it pulls time and space, and projects and magnifies thought. It refracted the thoughts one had inside to realization. What bonds, what bloody press dragged into being the perihelion? Although I have constructed the tower around it I have been given the freedom to interpret as I see fit. Moments in time. I define my deeper emotions as feelings. Sentimentality is the narrowing of experience to an emotionally familiar where misty value expands, like the majesty of an ivory tower rising from the fog, delicate delineations of previous patterns of chance. The past unalterably determines our journeys in the present. The essence is that if life and co-incidence are harmonious then one follows a synchronous labyrinth so that life is time's fool and thought life's slave and we surrender to time; order in movement. However just as order is not such an advantage as a sense of chance can lead to different points of perspective, so time is only our name for the motion of consciousness. It is a convention. She stays in her ivory tower when she should be reaching for spontaneity through the perihelion. Where once was wax the candle shows its hairs.

The creepers, the large wailing ships, were darker in the water today. This evening there was little but shapes and Adam apples of long agents to re-affirm him. Like a pen pal in queries of lust for what was not there, he rounded the fourteen planks to the dull, thudding and ominous calls of the junk-jetty. Reeking, echoing pipes where misplaced cargoes were dumped and rehandled spoke to him of the ugliness, the emergence of decay, of pops and clicks and…pigs "…Pig haul, pig haul!" The rough metal turned into pink and black pummelling flesh for a second, the squeals, the attention of the shipmates; then plunged into the water followed by a shipmate. Live cargo turned under the hull of ships Ned thought. He scampered down, collars up, dull hazy lights, sharp points of light, murky coldness and liquid softness. Polluted icy breezes cloaked his body in what could be described as a street corner pose from his father's day. A voice of Rita Caprita, the siren of the docks, called from the gangplanks above:

"Come show me your company, come show me who you be". Ned lingered in the face of this femme fatale and his Christian egotism. He gazed towards the giant dishes where messages or impulses found radar connections and yet like an elephant pulse they were bloodied, thick matted memory. Ned's dreams were scattered with the illusion of time. Entry into diary of Ned Wood. When one drifts on a tide of half forgotten realities, peoples' hopes and fears, honour and respect as one, then pain is the hope. Wrapped up in a tightening tourniquet, the wound is bathed in vitriol to keep it open. For it is our hope. I often dream that I am on a coastal path, with the sins of the ocean washing around me tears in my eyes, players around me, pleasure and attention seeking. We know that there is a world in which we belong that draws on the insanity of those whose dreams have been overcome by the ocean of sin. British expression wrapped up in centuries of metempsychosis. Most people have abandoned the root I am after but I gather tinder wood in my dreams and light a fire of their hopes. Their dreams moss coloured phobias; treacherous and trendy I swing upward like a purple old grief shirt to wrap his childhood faith arms around a love I chose to lose and climb the cliff. Time was a howling woman there to hear what fear was out of my inside. I scratched and screamed upwards to flee as the tide brings in the working day. She shows me the bitten moon in the morning. We decide in the realm of reality surrounding the myth that we have imaginary thoughts from somewhere far more mysterious- have we been so seduced by the modern world that we fail to see the spectre of time? It is time that the tale were told of how you took a child and made him old.

Around the unholy docks he was becoming anxious, confronted by this spectacle of darkness, heralded by the moon which boomed round to control a ball, stationary before bouncing and hung like a lemon on L.S.D., craters in the sea of tranquility winking. There was a stirring in the womb of an adolescent while its orbit controlled the tide, and the moon swept to provide permanence in change. He was thinking his way through the fear and so Ned spoke, caught in the web of anxiety. "I loved innocence more than health or beauty, preferred her to the light since her radiance never sleeps. In her company and at her hands riches are not to be numbered. We renew the bearing of time as we sanctify our waves of conscious change to the beat of radar logic, and mediate a contagious feeling akin to gravity. We stand endowed with this power while the winds of change consume the land. We accept perception of time through coincidence and only radiate spirit to be persuaded again by logic to accept our progress as natural."

"And why deliver mine eyes from tears and my feet from falling. I will walk before the Lord in the land of the living. I believed and therefore will I speak, but I was sore troubled and said in my haste mine eyes see but lies... I think of the different ways I had to make you mine, why are you so far away, more than you'll ever know".

He felt less fearful and valued the naked existence of her connection. The raven headed woman jangled her keys provocatively. Her reflection beckoned to him to join her. Ned spoke: "My resistance reveals my nature, and it is strange to me that beauty is often slain in the depth of night." The woman pulled her hand through her hair and sighed

"Then you are a monster of Frankenstein's" she exclaimed neurotically and continued to rant in low, soft tones, "a passing complexion, watery eyes like dun-white sockets, and straight black lips...." as she melted into the shadows. The plateau of beauty's attraction led to an effect on Ned; not compliancy, not hometown friendliness but contradiction. Was he ugly, misshapen in this inky blackness?

The ruby misted third party disappeared and left Ned's walk strangely vacant as he walked by the river. Old father Thames carried on the same like the process of time from tributaries to the sea. Never to be turned back. Ned dipped his hand in, and simple ripples surfaced as arcs from the present, the pattern of the labyrinth emerging from the water. He heard from the gangplanks the woman talking faintly to another man. Well she has now gone, he thought and he thought of her eyes lighting up; and well she would. A cloaked figure stood beyond him and Ned felt an icy shiver engulf him like he used to feel on watching Doctor Who as a child.

Ned's feeling went to a cobweb on the Albert Bridge; the spider shuddered with a patient and deadly art. Nostalgia- the purpose seeded in time like a thought. I suppose we identify with it through assurance without a cause for feelings witnessed in others. Nostalgia can bring an obsession to the fore but the only way to rid yourself of it is to yield to it. Withhold it and it festers and grows inside you. Yield and it becomes the edgy side of your love, withhold it and it becomes immoral guilt.

He was engulfed in sorrow but he made up his mind that to plunge from the bridge would not be to sink but to soar. He turned towards the banks of the Thames, imitating the lagging gait of a cloaked man seeking to kill time. His notice was taken by the second hand books displayed on the parapet and was at the point of bargaining for a Balzac novel *The Wild Ass's Skin* when he noticed an inscription- *To daddy with love from Michael.* A smile of hope lit his face, and slid from his lips to his eyes like the flame on the remnants of a newspaper in the embers of a fire.

He felt as though Sian was here in his labyrinth, on the silent bridge across the Thames. Albert bridge by torchlight, the world sees her legend in their shop fronts as light imitation of another season to end the sweep of Oarystes' pride as if counting success over separation, held in their swanlike hands. But love is strange.... It cast his mind from the water to the sky and he noticed the brilliance there. He heard a piercing scream from the docks but the wind turned it to a melody. He thought the web shivered with sin, the sin of creation, and he was reminded the theme was a tender, still there and stranded path through which we finger a sense to hysteric cobwebs that were born to be together and raised her eyebrows, mingling with circumstance that perhaps we were part of the masters' plan. Her minuet breath to shiver the core in conversation of a perfect world, from the eve of prouder caverns to the open harbour front of afternoon, wholly there and deciding to manifest adolescence in equinox for the natural charm she seeded in the broken web to strike the sky with an acorn was never closed over her palm.

Entry in diary of Ned Wood As the gliding seagulls beat down on me, I looked upon the web core in exile and by torchlight it appeared to hide your words on enthusiasm, confidence and flimsy compromise because if love could fly it'd be caught in the web, as romantic as discerned, weary of interiors like Yamamoto: so when we had ground beauty to dust, for all we know, we did know, redemption. The spider carried on silently, but his song remained the same, hanging from a silver thread

Ned guided his perihelion to the bridge's roundabout: a forking of ways. Which of the five ways of the b.e.a.s.t. will you choose through the resolution of the perihelion? belonging, evil, ardor, spontaneity or truth. It was a secret wind behind the brain, a sphinx of light which sat on the eyes, the skull, the cells, the cabined ears holding forever the code of stars as the secret night descended. It was the wisdom of ancient astronomy. It was what Ezekiel called a stone of fire. This prism had seen into the sky.

To predict the solstices and paths of the killing moon; monuments and myths mirroring the code of stars in heaven.

He caught sight of a man shaving in the window opposite and thought of his countenance and his desperation. Both fought the shadow caught in the mirror. A crowd, a wave of life's contours descended on him, face not free from rat nor mask. He saw himself as they saw him, trapped by destiny, divisible in the confusion and as every musical transference of the crowd defined a confused harmony, he thought of his body as it took the strain; tendons of such thinness supporting wiry strength condoning acceptance. He joined their conspiracy. This was a membranous perihelion flying in the face of airstreams: magnifying and raising to a point of vector resolution a half-buried conscience to attain nebulous confident pulses, directing hidden messages to adoption mode. Love can tell you what you want to hear but in the same breath she can steal, that's why his love for Sian didn't come easy. Ned accumulated visual completeness in an anatomically correct continuum moving to the contours of the crowd whose facets had been imprinted on him: he felt safer as an individual: drifting capillaries ignited, wavelength and weight converging, he escaped through the gates of a church and left the crowd behind him, not free from rat nor mask.

Ned saw the graves whose clawing ancestry gave him the perspective of going by the book, a book with a rose on every page and his rose tonight was the coincidence, like a costumeless bather at noon, of Sian sitting eating oranges, her white skin camouflaging her with the gravestones. Extract from diary of Ned Wood. In this wry child of honesty I saw the very sign of the sunrise of power and intellect, in the fun and genuine compatibility, in the offer of help I call caution, in the countenance, the nemesis of devotion, symmetry, traditional values and exertion she portrays…time. "I see we are both making our way through the graves"

"When we slice into this living world, maybe" as she turned the knife towards him "I am sore for what I never bore; the openness which was easily found and augmented into a different hope when it ought to have impacted the hurt that rusts inside my head to the dance of the leaves"

"You need to have hope", replied Ned

"Just when you have achieved your hopes they go and attach themselves to something else and the process stars all over again. How many wounds will open before the first blood falls: life's a bitch and then you die" and she claimed these words as her own, but he'd heard them said a hundred times, maybe less, maybe more.

"All their lives, their loves-it seems so sad". They looked around the pale grave-strewn yard and a chill reached into her heart. The lightening struck in the blackness. He felt as though they had lived before: their purpose seemed as hallowed and fragile as only destiny is. He believed they could touch the whole winding sigh of England, through a ticket dropped in the cat's cradle-wise smile. He handed her a letter he had written that afternoon.

"Your hair divine, your voice like wine from the depths of the city, echoes between leafy glades, between the town sways, where time and mystery lie", she read aloud. He looked into her eyes.

"The space between the orbs is a consuming passion but that does not mean that I am a consumer who just buys into the faint-at-her-beauty dream." He was lying. In this world of image generation, where beauty was bought and sold, or just played back on video, he felt as though he was looking not buying into the whole dream- the motorbike, the beautiful woman, and take my breath away playing in the background; the attitude that sits on a silver cloud saying never enough. He was, however, as hooked on the paradigm of beauty as anyone, predictably enslaved.

"Love is too mysterious to realize, too simple to behold. Love lies inside you and yet you search from my feet to the horizon- as if you have all the time in the world"

"From my ivory tower I have, for you are the sweet deer of youth. I'm still a lot like the past when our love for the inside like a deer the quickest flew-

"Do we view the world from an ivory tower?"

"I can't help but look at you through false hope as I linger on your jaunty brown eyes" Their eyes met and something mysterious passed between them.

"Looks are deceiving so you had better beware things that you see aren't necessarily there", she said embarrassed. He turned to get up but Sian was already gone, through the rain that fell and drifted on the crisp air. She drove her deux château to get away from Ned; I must say I can sympathize, to find some kind of happiness.

Ned returned to his room, bedraggled, and one might say he had a long time in the grave to think of her, still he turned to part of her he did possess –the picture of her. It hung in natural shadow in a pose, which chose to reveal white skin underneath soft flowing fabric and the motion of youth was captured there. Her shingled black hair would cascade onto her shoulders in tight spirals if she let it. The breeze had stolen a strand or so of her hair and he knew that her expression would last awhile when it seemed like forever in the first place, for her lips rested in the promise of a smile, as if she had seized the opportunity to tell him that it takes nothing to be natural. Neither accepting gravity or starlight- Ici l'enfant du paradise.

Ned clung to the potential of science, pulling mans' world of the heart with mechanical simile ruling under the emotion. He had a thin film of certainty by which his body achieved contact in his mind. Man is hypotentional in all but dreams and when you rule the dreamland you will hide in dreams to never go back to where people don't care. He would not be told that he suffered from moodswings but when he felt manic he would vehemently deny it, and when depressed he would not care. He lived for the stoke. The memories of joy, which would enhance his mood and connect himself with her. She had saved his life from misery but had given him havoc. The sleeping all over the world screamed. He turned his thoughts to unceasing sleep of what he had always been his very essence. Loneliness. Thus dreams took hold.

"Well you might as well call it love man, cos if you got it today you don't wear it tomorrow and as we found out on the train tomorrow never comes." Futuristic dream puke. Sian stared out from her cave at the erupting dreamscape. Her raven cawed unkindly at the havoc. In the room of forking ways destiny found himself hesitant to which of the five ways he will choose. He lay transfixed by her beauty, waiting for when she would come round, when he knew then that his collection of heaven would be treated with active scorn, the innocence of his accomplishments with felicitous force. Out of longing he knew that great wonders have been won.

As he viewed her smile; dry, wry and delicate as a thousand finite obligatory equations; but open, enigmatic and animated with the closeness with which she treated people, he turned the disparity of his thoughts over to her and was clear in his conviction that there was no algorithm, which could describe such beauty. Ned shifted his weight from one side to another, and silently mulled over her words upon seeing it- a face to scare the pigeons. He mused upon being the last pigeon to go and smiled at the thought she would have – so stupid as to beggar belief he would prefer to be trodden down than to fly. The body of sorrow floated upon the surface of the heathen soil as the firm ground turned the pigeon to sludge.

We see rise the secret wind behind the perihelion, thoughts splitting light five ways of the b.e.a.s.t. as the storm circled and the sky whimpered and moaned. Ned was reading the dog-eared book, the Wild Ass's Skin and thrashed and called out as if caught in a dilemma. "Which of five ways inside my heart" said the sorceress? A storm was brewing and it brought the two together separated by distance, now separated by seconds. She read a poem to calm her and, awoken by his unease, he busily scribbled one in his diary whilst they both watched the ensuing fireworks

Love's first promise ignites the heavens
Thunder peels to the white host in the sky
Fine rays of inspiration electrify
The course of racing clouds to evaporate
Heighten your spontaneity
La spontanete crainture des caresses

Love's second promise aroused Electra's desire
Sometimes if we freefall from reality
We place hooks in hilarity
And reel out their silken chord
To comfort and expand from fun to honesty
Through your life like a storm.

All influence is someway immoral
Because life is self discovery
Old man rain's livery spells that the only way
To rid temptation is to yield to it
Like a cloudless innocent day
That is swept away by the storm

Chapter 3 With These Eyes Before

Ned had decided to live in this godforsaken Essex town because it had a 24hour, themed casino. It was the Mecca of Essex for anyone who was interested in gambling and this night, as the storm diminished; Ned was drawn to it, rising out of the forest, shrouded in mist. Blithely in the battle for cultural merit the Egyptian-themed casino was king. It was part of the view from the ivory tower that made him deal in what was not reality, in obsession. It was an hour of pleasure, during which his thoughts freed him from misfortune but is there a less pleasing thing in the world than obsession? His present woes give the lie to his hopes; yet he looked to the future, which was not his, to indemnify him for these present sufferings. Pleasure was as fleeting as the fluttering of bank notes in the hands of the croupier who handed him his chips, setting upon his actions the weakness of his nature. The gamblers nodded with a pull of the lifted hand, the voice of the croupier with vested comprehension. An inner materialization followed (that contemplation is for losers); a sweetness of surprise mixed with the heady contentment of a friend followed a win. Every bet placed entombed a shattered flower and there was a metaphor of indifference in love's second fever- the moon quits the sky he does not love.

Where the fantasy was the seed the dream had gone but the casino was real, the crowdedness of the room subsided as space beckoned him, a gent bayed like a wolf, the male nature showed through, seedy, dividends to be gathered begetting forms of divisibility, insight and snooping like wax trapping a hair. Gambling was not reality but in the labyrinth of chance...Ned observed the way people moved, like wolves stalking. The gents and their bitches feigned and swooned, lady grinning souls illuminated your existence a mere hair's width. The gauntlet of eyes were concentrated on one table where an Italian had lady luck. Ned went straight up to the table, and, as he stood there, flung down a piece, which he held in his hand, without deliberation. Lady luck rolled it onto the black, though anyone but a new hand would have divided his money into three parts to give himself more chance. "Make your game... The game is made... bets are closed" and with each eagerly fixing his eyes on the prophetic wheel, Ned was held there until the wax melted and he was free: "Even! Red wins." The ivory touched the chip with a little click, as it swept it with the speed of an arrow into the heap before the bank.

    ...."Then speak of one who loves not wisely and not well..." The conversations continued around him, a bitch yawned as the candle sings, a slow softness followed as he found a corner and lit a cigarette gently as a breeze to trouble heaven. His emotions on what was really there, hinted like a sly smile on the face of a girl. He almost took the role of a redeemer of any remorse found, his paranoia coming to the fore to sympathize with these gamblers. It is true that even though you lose 3000 if you win 300 you are hooked. He was on a losing end and so he took his winning smile and a flier and walked into the street with no reason won; like the gravity of a pamphlet's rhetoric. He tramped through the discarded pamphlets, stirring in the wind as though they were alive, and the trail led on like a wax heart pulling the hair of the labyrinth to the forest surround.

It was dawn. Four strong winds that run lonely, he thought as a jogger caught his view. What were these people, he thought, who get up for a run before work? Car parks, bottles and cutlery greeted him before he could make it to the woodland. The cockroaches molded in the ground, the moths shivered in the air, mushrooms crushed into view as animals disappeared from it. The place was less of a wilderness than a vacuum, Ned tripped over it. The Hoover looked misplaced and in a sci-fi dream could have appeared the bloody remnants of a robot war; then again he was in no mood for a war he thought as he felt that pang of guilt, which had led to the robots taking arms against an uncaring human race. He chanced upon the volume control in his Walkman and decided it doesn't become his mood to mull over the human rubbish so he continued until he watched a stranger appearing from out of her home. He felt a little voyeuristic but watched silently as the surrogate sister stooped and picked up a leaf. "Sian's name is like morning mist, a taboo, a sanctuary as I pop her Ariel rings skimming o'er the grove to sustain the heartier resin apart the clouds, in early morning reverie of the nocturne and blonde."

Down the pub she surveyed him with a look which said I'm uneasy because of something you've done, whilst he just gently squeezed the life out of his pint and wondered if he would spiral any lower, but by this time her conversation had switched to well developed butchers, her shrill laugh braking him out of the unease she portrayed earlier. The rest of the pub continued to act out the Guinness advert and the talk was going cheap. Ned was always taking on board other peoples realities she had shyly once told him and he thought about this until he realized that he was being choked at the ankle by a small dog and thought that maybe he should start acting tougher.

The cider breeze saturated his spirits and made despair out of the languor of the dry morning. It reminded him that providence was strength and those things along the way: company, steady employment, riches, relationships were as incidental to the changes he was going though, traveling through the middle of the bloody perihelion. Amidst the trees and pacing the pathways vigorously he noticed the blood-color of his best shoes. Strange, he thought, but his depression was compounded by the closeness of the vegetation, wandering lost in a forest full of painful vagaries, looking again at the tightness that stretched at his navel to the skeletons of trees. Drenching logs could drag away the shapes, the crooked billets; the stray monoliths of an ancient wood, which fed the silence. Suddenly the silence was broken by a hollow drawl of ulterior cords emerging from the lips of a girl moving amongst the trees some way ahead but disappeared amid the air of hallowed mirth like Sian leaving the graveyard that night. Now as then it would avail the shadowy specters, the moss shields and crooked Lenore of their indignant ghost to float out of the damn earth and Ned had to steady himself not to think that the floating voice was a ghost's, as he passed the spiral tree.

Extract from diary of Ned Wood We all have our own style from the tuning of the light of reason from expressions shared and arcs of imploring; the only things that resist when sanity fails and one is stripped to the bone. The subtle cognitive call of a pigeon heralds the spiral tree's magic and hides in the quality of lichen; the shades and transience of pagan influence. Memory. For I go mournfully so she may fear no wrong, fin de ciecle as vivid, deep and durable as the illusive closeness of desperation. Imprinted, imposing patterns emerging from the character of daisy lead to the spiral tree; now in front of him covered in mossy green. Ned touched its bough. He felt its life and a peace like his mother telling him the story of the faraway tree as a child permeated his spirits.

Media opened to the atmosphere, he read the story of a woman who was found without her eyes: jealousy, he read was the suspected motive. The perpetrator was called the eye trophy killer and had left a swathe of destruction through East London. It was Rita Caprita, a butterfly lavishly laughed at the heavy air while bees at environmental stress looked for eyes to gouge out amid the flowers. Do they beam down worst upon women, he thought, and was jealousy distinct to the victor's spoils? The shortfall, natural as the vain camouflage of spiraled, fearsome beauty ingrained under a leafy glade, would be a nursery rhyme to the sky. Perhaps there was an angry pixie, Silky, moonface and the saucepan-man in some other–worldly dimension he thought as he dreamt. In the faraway tree from which all things stem and find harmony and return, the five ways of the b.e.a.s.t. find a balance. As he climbed the tree to reach the land of birthdays at the top he found himself, as a rule always furiously independent, becoming part of the forest world from which man had come. His hands had turned to bark, his feet of clay, his face of leaves and his limbs of wood. The primeval flora in its teeming glory, the great water spirits, the zephyrs of the air, and the life giving sun awoke his senses- he was the green man from which we all spring. In the land of birthdays at last the roots of life inhabit.

Ned woke up rested and replenished and noticed the surrogate sister standing by him balancing on the upturned, half-buried Hoover in the woods. "You know your so petty don't you and spiteful. You kind of hid the fact that your personality was a napping, stupid sod who cares for nothing or no-one. No don't- you're ill-informed as mud you selfish sod". Ned remembered he hadn't rung her since they both collided like flotsam on a beach one evening. Sex was a lovely thing you're looking for but it is a bit like a little child locked out of the room when it doesn't go right. "Many guys have designs from a hole but your avoidance only goes to show that you are stuck in a very deep one". She was obviously upset but he could only remember fragments, as it was a drinking session thing.

"Yes" he said stumbling for words "I remember that you were a socket for Jesus and I was your love cable".

"Well I just thought I'd tell you that you are wasting your time that's all- oh and if you want any more services of a physical nature you can bloody well..." and with that she fell from her precarious balance and her head smashed on the ground from her more than ample height. Not even a scream was unleashed on the fading sky. She was motionless, silent.

"Well that's pricked the eyes of contention" Ned was not being sensitive. "Come on are you alright" he exclaimed as he knelt by her. One of her eyes was hanging by a thread and she had had her head embedded in the corner of the vacuum. "Jesus" exclaimed Ned; then a strange thing happened; he reached down and plucked the eye from its socket! As he looked at it and the rare beauty, a sensation of phantasmagoria engulfed him. The eye was perfect, so delicate an orb of priceless purity. He said something aloud "quid si coelem ruat" even though he knew not what it meant. He felt an intense feeling of possessiveness he had not felt except over Sian and the feeling he had stifled all this time suddenly impacted upon him. He stretched to his full height and wrapped the still dripping eyeball into a hanky and slipped it into his pocket. At that he looked around at the scene of morbid putridity, he left slowly but soon aware that the trees shielded his every move, he fell into a euphoric nonchalance and ran through the concealing forest, back home with his macabre prize.

Chapter 4 Morning Shone Youthful

He sat in his chair and while making a cup of tea he fingered the handkerchief, feeling a centered tranquility he had not felt in a long while. He held the cup in his hand; the thought of its prevalent symmetry forming orbs in his mind, the tea at a gentler stage of candescance seeped leeward from its pot. The radial symmetry traced by the milk into an oval cup, calmed the frugal remnants of his sanity. Needs must fly he thought. He did not feel grief though perhaps the absence of feeling; he felt fascination.

"Tis past that melancholy dream- the joy of her desire by morning shone, by night concealed" he chanted, for he now possessed something tangible, something worthy of this mortal coil- he could now linger on her metempsychosis. He had no human fears, no force of time had she. He shuddered at the thought but meanwhile the fascination was at work urging him ever forward to use his emotions. I scrape through resin to a starry bone and a blood perihelion...the handkerchief revealed its prize and the rarity of the workmanship was clear, just as mists cleared, so the hidden strength of colour like wings aglow unfurling the whole drama of the world dawned on him. The fractals of the iris sparking like cameras was the beauty existing within it but there was more than that; as he brooded on it, it became crystal clear that the eye provided the essence of what the vampires in his dream coveted; everlasting youth.

Sian had lain on Walpurgis night with a sorceress's view of the stars, the hex Ned had cast leaving a print of the Milky Way upon the lids of her eyes. She dreamt preparing to right the wrongs of old; for she had cried the tears of the mighty oceans and seen the print of stars in heaven. She had a dream where she was a saint, her voice like divinity. Blotting out the transgressions, as a thick cloud she pieced together redemption; "Though their sins be scarlet, they be as white as snow, though they be red like crimson, they are as wool!" she spoke. She felt as though the tears of the devil had burnt the seeds of pity and the radiation led her to the heart of a burning church. She was howling at God for the ones that got left behind. "Oh mine eyes are ever towards the Lord because he shall pluck my feet from the net; look thou upon me, have mercy upon me, for I am desolate, afflicted and in misery" she spoke in the guise of holy martyrdom.

Sun streamed in from the French blinds onto a reclining figure and in an air of suspended permanence Sian's smile turned to an otherwise faint wish to get out of herself, lose herself, swinging majestically out like a brush through her hair. The timeless energy of her complexion engulfed her shameless brown eyes and her shingled black hair her complexion. Her figure was perfect and she curved to the lightness of being as her eyes opened to the world of her bedroom. Thais, the mistress of generals and wife of Pharaohs was so much duller than her. Too late to dream of sleep. How unbearable the whiteness of the blinds. She thought. Her majesty glanced wryly out of the sun drenched liturgy of a room as she felt complete in the thought of her love which had turned her art-deco world into a gathering of heavenly pace existing within the boundaries of her belief. She was instinct and reflection; a promise of something better than your wildest dream, the broad prosaic result of which is a mood of euphoria and inferiority; but not emptiness, filled by her shameless face. She knew instinct and reflection would cope elegantly with the loathing and love that characterizes our dreams and life.

Dear Ned

I sit and contemplate the past year and it's been exciting, uplifting- not strange or tedious as so many a year has edged. Yet so many good ideas have been lost in dreams and episodes of high society. My memory is bad and my patience dull. I feel as though I want to run from where I am and run from where I arrive. Italy I suppose. I wrote about your therapy sessions:

Naughty Men
Two smartly dressed men sitting opposite each
other at a desk. Dr A is sucking his thumb. He
takes it out of his mouth upon noticing the patient.
Dr. A :   Hello, can I help you?
Patient : Ah (laughs) I'm here to help you,
misterrrrr...?
Dr. A :   Doctor Roback, but you can call me Ken.

Patient : No, I'm Doctor Ken Roback
Dr. A :   (nodding knowingly, rubbing chin) Ah, I see – you think you're me.
Both :   Have you seen …(both men laugh; a second of silence)
Patient : Have you seen a psychologist?
Dr. A :   No, only my patients.
Patient : I really don't have time for this.
Dr. A :   Neither do I. © Kieron Hall

I was glad to receive your letter because even though persuasion doesn't count, affection does. I recognize so much angst among what were such innocent eyes. My boyfriend is staying in Syracuse and I haven't spoken to him in ages. I don't expect you're interested but there you are. I thought I'd write you a romantic poem Mr. Wood.

Let the web of time, define
Between the candle and the starlight
When passages turn into nights
And the lights grow dim
Nights turn into towers
And I throw at whim
My Eve's innocence
And look long past since
Bowler hat in a giant's cave
The flame who's hew is bent
To make our love shape
The mouth of wisdom sent.

Let the web of fate, elevate

Between the candle and the starlight.
Lets fly away tomorrow
A just assertion
Far from pain or sorrow
To a distant shore
Where the near meets the far.
Our souls tower
Bowler hat in a giant's cave
Of a stray dragon
Through the Milky Way
Like drips of conversation.

From the case spills his black cloak like a blackened bull. Stars glittering here and there, distantly in his warm hands he smelt the planet Mars, of iron and the planet Venus, a green ivy smell and the planet mercury, a scent of sulphur and fire and he could smell the milky moon, milky white and glowing with a light of its own. He put the eye into a glass jar. It plunged to the bottom and hung motionless. He tightened the lid, put it into his cupboard and was away to work, but he soon felt strangely morose. As he entered the village of Waterbeach, a murder of crows was staring at him by the airfield gate. He uttered a password to them thinking that they were guardians of the airfield, long memorized, as their breed were accustomed to be. A disturbing resentful smile formed upon his lips, unleashed from the sky like blood seeping from a wound. He suddenly had the picture of the girl falling in his head; the thin outward movement of her arms, the opus movement of her hips, the crushing momentum, and in her flesh the moment of her death seemed to him his conceit in keeping the eye; the conceit she shadowed him with seemed to come from the crows piecing stares and suddenly the purity of the bridge to metempsychosis he kept while with the talisman of the eye seemed less steady. The pinprick of guilt pervaded his thoughts as he read from his newspaper- local girl found dead. No suspicious circumstances except that an eye was supposedly taken by crows. Verdict misadventure. The crows were beating down on him and he had joined their deceit as he read on. The eye trophy killer had sent in an article, which criticized the spineless, sickening reliance that the modern world had instilled. As Ned read on it reminded him of his favorite band, Strangelove of dark, brooding humor that instilled its own tradition.

Folding the paper to his side Ned felt disturbed. The danger was that he was being drawn closer to the trophy and further from reality. It would take the willful goodness of Sian's personality to bring him from this brink. The sorceress was to hold out her staff as he stumbled in the darkness and keep his feet from slipping. Sanctuary from these feverish smiles. The sorceress had let her raven go from her crossbow and like a vision on a raw October day wrought a miracle of flashing and dipping low in savage flight. Suddenly Ned's heart sang as the Dakota brilliantly banking, lit up the scene in a display contrasting to the haughty static grace of the sorceress. It flew above like corn comes green pulls back the years. The sorceress was able to transcend truth and run by devious paths to the old seeds of wonder. The noisy engines whirred and buffeted the breeze. Ned felt calm; the crows were just a comical group of overeager carrion after all. As the Dakota loomed overhead he felt cozened by the dull hum of the shadow passing him over.

He worked for Peter at a company called Aces High. They kept old aircraft flying for filming and air shows. Ecology is innocence and Ned often believed in his work that he was Icarus. The error lay in the boy's lack of respect for the nature of his materials- wax. He flew too near to the sun, which isn't a safe or friendly place for wax to be. His mistake wasn't in trying to fly. That comes with the territory of being a human. His problem was an inability to take seriously the essence, or being-ness of the natural ingredients with which he worked.

The wing was in pieces, and the afternoon began by scrutinizing for conservation or renewal by dye penetrant inspection. A discarded air gun lay on the floor hissing. They used preventative maintenance on the planes as a whole if they could, based on the original data books. Ned settled into his work and the hours went past. It was a perfect place, an airfield surrounded by a patchwork of fields in a small village in Essex. It had been a squadron base until the 60's and still smelt of the past; Ned took his mask off and surveyed the officers' bar. Tainted glass hid beneath wraiths of cobwebs mocking the pains so that their faded glory shone green and pink in the autumn sunlight. A hint of hallowed virtue sat behind them, as if the faces of long gone RAF officers were peering up at the sky above, and made a feeling rise up in Ned of a green and pleasant land; for if the buildings and tarmac could talk, they'd be the gravity of time.

Twenty-six years earlier Michael looked up at the imposing black Dakota. As his eyes followed its majestic lines, it seemed to usher out an era. Underpinning his very reaction was his joys of standing with his back against the old stonewall watching the ensuing display. The tarmac squealed and fuselage buffeted against the wind as the Dakota flew down to land like a raven

But Ned was not Michael. Even as the fog continues to lie in the valleys, so does ancient sin cling to the low places, the depressions of the world consciousness. Despite his rage he still stumbled along in the fog of the void. The fog was the trimmer, sleeker, slimmer folk pouring drinks at the bar ruled by methods of control under the ethos of ignorance, counting little pennies from heaven to defend their physicality. He was susceptible to other people and his mood was overly affected by them. When you become a siphon for the world's sin, low esteem, drugs, interference from professionals, inference of these working types, materialism, vampirism and prejudice like criminality, madness, racism or nationalism, all the kings' men and all the kings' businessmen couldn't put him together again.

Ned tried to piece together the remnants of his reasoning to form a whole. He dealt in definites, which he could perceive, like innocence, nostalgia and scientific laws. He had made a fantasy world of perception to overcome his faults. The ways of the b.e.a.s.t. refracted thoughts he knew he had always had to realisation. Man's inhumanity to man continued his desolation; for one only has to step out into the void to find that man is still vulnerable. Belief is strength but it is important not to live in ignorance under a closed circle of belief. Tradition is a constant and the profanity is change and hence madness profane. There was a mad man who lived in a mad mad town and rode a mad horse; madly. The mad are pilloried as being wicked when it is the accusing, manipulative, incessantly selfish people that are the threat. She was just so innocent, in many ways but also worldly wise. Give me time to open up my eyes. Extract from diary of Ned Wood. Innocence was a bid to stay safe, the actions of a shy teenager who sits next to a girl he fancies unsure of which way to go, thoughts rushing through his head but too shy to talk to her; a resolute fear called the awkwardness of exchange which was meant to disappear in conversation. Fears that led him to stay silent at parties were something he had eased himself out of over the years. Remember the awkwardness, the impotence, the panic, the inexperience, the emphasis on yourself but it didn't last long: it was just a memory of putting you on a pedestal while other men put you on the pill.

The letter was on the mat when he got home, and an aberration of the heart freed him from his musing as he opened it, recognizing the handwriting instantly. Seated with the letter Ned felt a sense of accomplishment; therein the insecurity for love that had brought him thus far which wreathed his movement with an emptiness, and ate at him like barbed wire and maggots, disappeared like tension. It was a sanctuary to seat the light of her years for the messages of his heart and it captured his thoughts. He lit a candle and held up the jar for a reaction of the eye. It danced in the light to steady his nerve for each new tomorrow, holding him as youth feeds the innocent abandon. Real end solutions kept coming forward from the facets of the iris; a settling, dreamier world to the one, which greeted his reality; like a chemical, which encouraged his flights of fancy, fathoming his darkest secrets. It enhanced the perspective he had, and conjured up true and meaningful admiration for Sian. It was the vehicle of chance in the labyrinth. For he saw through the eye perihelion a sign not to go quietly, or go by the book and stick with his loneliness, but would embark on a mission to slip into bed or something with a future that Sian belied, sworn to continue in fear, love and hope five different ways, where dreams are never enough.

His body cut a circuit on his bed. Sleep deprivation made the cool air turn hot and he felt the fire in the wild wind or saw walls burning bright coloured air. Castles burnt in the forest of his mind and called him to action. His reply was written before he had taken his coat off, and typed it up because his handwriting was atrocious. He had the ideal opportunity to invite Sian to Sicily with him on board the Catalina. He and Peter were to fly it to Syracuse that month. The opportunity was a godsend and he looked at the eye in exhilaration. His talisman had done a marvellous job. He had a sweet, malevolent, nurturing symbolism in his head; a solace of a vulnerable soul growing. He only wanted her safe conduct through her delicate framed world; to be his for an afternoon. In his mind she stood there in fond embrace like she had re-established laughter but first he had to get some sleep. Ned fell into a deep contented sleep.

A huge ray of fire had struck the ground. Out of this ground a spiral tree emerged. Iduna, the goddess of love, had an apple fixation and she had heard that the tree bore golden apples. In the gods, the penny colour of Iduna led like an apple of youth fruiting along the dairy path. She was tricked by the god Loki under the influence of the vampires of the earth. She came to earth under the late summer moon, among the stone circles, in view of the meteor's crater. "Daughter to the stars" said Loki, "chase the meteor's bloom, red set with explosives where there is an apple of gold, thrown and crumpled to kinship".

As Ned saw her he was in rapture. The twinkling of the stars, love divine, together throughout time, crossed his path forever. She was precious to the gods and carried the secret of their youth in her casket of apples. To a motion fingered by fermenting shells vampires crossed the oceans. As they swam into the night, aware of Iduna's laced casket, the moon shone down. They swooped down and stole the casket of apples from Iduna. The gods were angry and grew old. The comet, which had streaked the earth with fire, and the strange alien tree that had grown from its charred remains, had caused the gods anger.

The vampirism sect who had always coveted the gods' youth begun to worship this tree. Ned, with the other mortals, thought of his mortality, listening to the strange music of the vampires who were holding vigil there and thought that the most important things in life were the things that you got away with from the gods. A strange sensation gripped him, as if he were taken over by a malevolent force. He was aware that there was a realm beyond the senses in which we endure the elements in life, all tied together into a labyrinth of malevolence. Death is so close to us that the distance between it and the life centre inside us cannot be measured but has become something external, held further away from us every day. Like an unobtainable apple of youth.

Chapter 5 The Boat of Venus

The Catalina was standing picturesque and majestic against the grey sky and green fields, looking like a spruce goose in the paddock waiting to fly. The duration of the sun had passed and their feet broke the pallid runway dust as they approached. The black carrion were stepping sideways and buffeted by the wind they seemed not at all ominous today. Peter stood with a grimacing smile on his lips that pointed to an acquired knowledge. He knew the tracks, and stood pondering over the information in the charts as he wiped his sleeve over the black hull. Peter climbed inside and in his way he announced his misunderstanding of the elliptical screen to his right. He knew however that the ghosts of the past were waiting expectant and their valour seeped into him- as he was the only one who had flown the Catalina over the seas in its role as a torpedo amphibious aircraft. He bestowed his timorous knowledge with a fixed prejudice of one who had flown before.

Ned took the plane to his heart as he had done since they begun restoring it five years previously- he clasped its ruinous beauty to the burning in his soul. It had his expertise in its innards; the cabling and the control surfaces were his work. But he had the journey to revel in and as Sian stepped into the belly of the plane and sat in the bubble in the middle he was content as he could be. As he looked down elevation her brown eyes, the rule on the rise, overwhelmed him but as she listened to its history in precise detail, he saw that she held it in the same respect as he did. As the rush of the engines started Ned saw her fingers clasp the rail and dug russet into her hands. However the girl called patience soon recovered her doubt as the plane flew from the tarmac, the hull gliding bold and ravenous into the air.

It is difficult to describe flying because it is a feeling and sensation and from feeling to a purpose all of its own. To track a clearer vision is often to sound like you earn a commission on selling the sky. It opened his heart with no compare and pain and regret trickled away like the evaporating mist on the widows. Inside the womb of the plane they had a great view, the reconnaissance role of the plane giving a varying view of up to 360 degrees from the glass observation bubble. Peter sat by the cockpit, watching the trace element on the radar screen. Sian conjected that he looked responsible. Encouraged the pilot went into the thinness of thinnest of manoeuvres on the stick and clumsily the plane banked, abandoning the view of the ground with the sky heaving broad and the passengers stretched and basked in the afternoon sun above the clouds. Emotions tumbled like the clouds they left beneath them.

"No matter how far you have come, you always have further to go" Peter said: all were lost for words but their smiles shone through. A siren searched their novel approach to a motion fingered by fermenting violins as they flew into the distance aware of their laced firmament, emotions tumbling like clouds and Peter, the man we lost for words smiled elliptically from shoulder to shoulder in a winking and dramatic art. Sian glistened a half believing eye to Ned and lit up the scattered tallow in his receptive brain, reminding him he was flesh and bone, with indoor fireworks. Her stockings maladjusted his smile and he run for cover in his skull as he looked just like the poppy to the larkspur; embarrassed creating form from dark regions of sorrow quivering on the Living Earth Goddess spinning a tapestry of life. Love was telling him to stay; pperhaps the elegance of her form pportrayed the rapture of his heart, which she kindled and left him leering bleakly. Society is the pattern between the shibboleths we chase but she had helped him to find what was missing in society- his dreams. Flying became like a broken arrow to him which showed whenever the memory laps over the drag of the aircraft and countenance became the heart of man grafting a slow heading from the merriment and contentment of equity with nature to strike hammer purposed through the moving air like a propeller blade. Desperation and instinct drained a long sigh, holding their purpose flighty under the pale countenance and reflection.

Like Venus first held confidence with Vulcan, Sian sat communing with the rush of the engines, the wings cutting through the pressure of the air and nature's invisible art in the sky beyond them. She converted her psychic energies to the images and so came the imaginative, and the desired so that the forces within the cosmos; her achievements, qualities, belief, commitment and opinions flew in space and time like a small breeze lifted the craft heavenly toward the horizon. She wore content on her face. "There ain't nothing you can't do... and there is no connection between what is old and what is new...I could make a man out of nothing at all..." She continued in this vein for ages. Ned listened and thought she would have been trigger-happy if she'd have been in the war, but when he said this, she vehemently claimed she had a stealthy hand in all things.

He captured her expression in a photograph of glowing resonance. The fabric of their mandatory agreement covered any chagrin she had left for him. As the propellers beat in their ears like hornets wings she spoke

The fragile, transparent mist
Travelled 'neath wing
She swirled and she curled
On her way to the mill

The gulls marked time
By the sails that were turned
She, too powerful to be seen
Like the Lord God almighty

And we like the crushed grain
A product of her making
So easily undertaking
Enabling the body of Christ to rise

Those creaking sails keep sounding her fayre

The gull's whip is bare
And I breathe in purity © Lorraine Bearryman

Rustic of mind they emblazoned a trail over the countryside, the air shuddered and parted at their bow, and first one, then many a brow of a hill came and went. The lives of thousands of people were strewn on the ground beneath and they flew resplendent over them. The countryside of shepherds and windmills, which had been their home, was left far below them, and as Ned navigated a course that would take them over the beaches where he and Sian had first met- in two beach huts on the Essex coast, they had acclimatized to all those years ago, when she had stood like a statue, the white marble composing virtue consumed by waves, pounding upon his grave expression. For his soul; lay in the serf, where she placed her feet, like a faithful promise, incidental to their air-Bourne vision. Their heads bowed in passion's gaze, like spirit in movement. They passed over the Martello tower, which was the highest point either of them had been in the heady days of childhood innocence. "Do you remember building boats in the sand?" Ned asked.

"I remember waiting till the sea washed over us", replied Sian. They smiled. There was a bit of turbulence as they passed over the sea, as the offshore winds met them, but it diminished, their silhouette riding over the sea's olive-green surface below them. Rainbow swirls and parallels gave way to shifts and sweeps and fans, pastels to silver sparkling over it all; the crystal sea of a strange marine world that the Catalina was designed for awaited them.

Ned began to ply his wood curd dream, her sequined top shining like peacock feathers, of thick grain made, the closeness of his only love too much to bear. He ran for cover in the temple of love believing pain and remorse left behind by his talisman, the eye. He bowed his head too afraid of what he had to say. " Heavy ships are so lightly thrown by the sea." She was a testament to beauty and looked at him softly. "You are like sea mist, your lips the day has kissed, misty in your stare that holds my gaze so fair. Your mood of melancholy's despair, crumpled and drawn to kinship, tied with seafarers' rope- your secrets are like the sea flotsam revealing the night's ecstasy. Return her here to me so that there remains a forlorn hope."

"I fly the thoughts that are promised to the night, born in darkness and of starlight. The rule of silent lips to ease the hurt inside dips my tongue. Remember the wolf's den? Of beauty's risk and nature's air. It returns your face, your lips, your gracious stare." The motion brought them together and they kissed. The Catalina still rode the weather but inside the haven of the plane they were alone, slowly and gracefully kissing.

"For what is peace but to sleep with beauty? For eternity all is true: to fall on your brow tender and smooth. If it weren't for us wolves, lovelorn this far from heaven the sky would resound to the sound of a thousand of us, making love beneath the stars. For these are the riches of the poor- a bed and a starlight lover for sure"

"To Yeats the Delphic oracle was a sigh: and those who came upon the shore, even the tall Pythagoras soon lay there as well", she replied. They kissed.

"I try to frame my emotions but I may as well try to catch water in a net for the waters disclose my choice to feel as a small boy, lining his pockets with pearls, furled in harlequin blue, commemorating dreams of the sea." Ned's love was a love that was saved and yet it was her essence- power from the land, coincidence; a mischievous puck from some internal source, too beautiful to endure, too impossible to believe. Say the word mine, and it was gone. Colors flew away from him and then back again, normally lost in pallid wandering he felt a connection, which he took for granted she did too. They felt drawn, comforted. The plane forded a river with ease as they kissed. It showed them a thousand new words spoken in silence and verses that only ravens cry. Their minds were fixed but time and circumstance brought them together in metempsychosis of labyrinthine spirals.

"By an angel's wing you are thinking from your hideaway of a secret, guided ever to flow through the truth of humankind. You are precious and to all evidence an angel 'neath wings of feathers and chest of gold, plumes of hair 'neath halo of old. A triumph born in glory of love and honor. Endeavors to try your patience every now'n again. If it had been an angel's kiss, we'd fly over the sea majestic forever. A space between cabined ears; an angel in your eyes."

"The smell of you which brightness burns around me still. No greed no desire. I speak only to say: you can be anything you want. Every colour you are." Ned had seven views of France but saw only Sian's beautiful face and the chariots of angels were colliding as their wings of passion prevailed. The strands of her hair directed him into her arms. He had never believed in the existence of earthbound angels but looking at her he wondered if it were true. He laughed, he couldn't help himself and the smile walked away from him as she settled, but the passage of time wasn't actuality and they fell into a more passionate kiss binding their consciousness together in the realms of tiny sparking dreams. He believed in love and somehow he knew she did too. There was a coyote with small white feet. The same instinct as created order in the pack also left him in solitude, the symbol of aggression being the byword amongst the course silver ghostly beasts which roamed with impatience just as the wind howled, when he came near to a beautiful black wolf running free by a lake. He had no time to wonder, though wondrous it was. She had chosen him. The very sharpness of their breaths deluded the scene of mercy in a vulpine world. Eminence with the thrill and pleasure only love can bestow on the wild and forlorn. It was such that Ned felt as they passed over the icy mountains, where they roamed as wolves and for a while they made a meal of the wonderful despair they felt.

People said that she was easily led and they were half right. The friend Sian had conveyed was a passionate friend and a cheating heart is still a beating heart. He listened to his and hers as they breathed together. The fact that they were here at all felt like destiny. The weather was overcast but Ned's mood was flying as they passed over the Riviera and into the blue Mediterranean. The deep vibrant colours made them think of secluded bays and holidays. Confidence was valuable these days and for Sian this was really what it was all about. She said that was not sure of the things she cared about any more. This made Ned feel just a hint of pride but he was afraid that he had spoiled the balance she had found. She told him to mind affairs of the heart and, just like her mother said, the miliscention of wisdom is to compromise yourself sometimes. As the two souls had rushed together he looked more into her eyes than he had ever dared before and made a mental note that he would only give his opinion and his opinion was that it was hard to take from such grace though. He only knew that she had the cards he needed in her hand, and this did not amuse him.

"Must the cards all be dealt facing down?" He said after a while. Well, what else do you do but play cards to avoid the obvious wrapped up in coincidence. He had worn his heart on his sleeve, heedful of her attitude like a stain on his aim. But his aim was true. He thought of his fish at home and how he had forgotten to feed them. "Not again" he muttered and his thoughts started to become ever so slightly malicious. It is so common for passion to arouse a hidden jealousy and he thought- what if Sian fails to return his affection. What if she spurns his advances? He did not know whether he could cope with the passions she had aroused.

The clouds began to disperse as the plane soared into view of the coast and with a rush of the engines and some rolling they found a line of action parallel to the frothy sand of the coast. With trees and roofs finally in view after the sparseness of the sea, a very relaxed network of civilization was revealed. The vegetation was sparser here and there, and fields trimmed with lemon and almond trees appeared then disappeared on their trail. They were following the coastal railway in case of emergency procedures and because Ned had become weary of navigating.

Dusk had been and gone and though neither passenger had any sense of time, they had a false affinity now and her demeanour seemed too courteous towards him. There was awkwardness which neither of them mentioned when she read out the location of her boyfriend's campsite. Three miles south of Syracuse it was run by a strange rose beetle man, a burnt out relic from the sixties who played the role of interpreter to Ian, the aforementioned boyfriend. Apparently it was covered in wild flowers and had apartments which both pleased Sian. The rose beetles were just an added attraction. But the rose beetles seemed to Ned to spit out a venom with every word she finished as the glowing phantasm of their embrace, the awakening of the flesh, left him. Unquenched by growing doom, uncertainness forked and gulfed the embarrassment she harboured. Dumbness and affection, doubt and euphoria opposed each other, and though she swooned over-dramatically as he reached out to hold her hand on landing, out of the body of affection prized an inner light synonymous with innocence. I loved innocence more than health or beauty, preferred her to the light since her radiance never sleeps. In her company and at her hands riches are not to be numbered.

He emerged from their journey with a deep-set happiness after all, and the engine was noisy, miss-firing as the landing lights showed the dark water beneath the amphibious craft rise towards them. The buffeting was painfully slow to subside leaving skimming patterns of fans on the crystal waters they had touched. The wake of the craft symbolized what had passed and it ain't what the moon did. The future belonged to Syracuse, winking and glinting, ahead of them over the breakwater.

PART TWO: Metempsychosis

Chapter 6 The Trail of the Dead

The sanguine sunrise, with his meteor eyes, his burning plumes outspreading in the distance was their first sight of Syracuse. They sat down tired, after crossing a bridge and rounding the sea defenses, on a small beach, small, as it was beautiful. A question formed upon Ned's still lips but passed and was never told. It was as if they had spent a week of twilight hours as the sun broke russet over the far side of the bay and shone resplendent in their eyes. On one side lay a garden full of the chatter of birds and on the other the ocean heaving broad, seagulls swooping over where the Catalina was moored. The sea lapped at their feet like minions at the feet of a master for they felt grand after their momentous journey. In a reflective mood Sian read from a guidebook of the city and musing on the facts of its past, she looked just like a witch of Etna. Its emerald crags glowed in her beauty's glance through the green splendor of the water's edge, while constellations were still dancing like fireflies in her folded palm. She had a wisdom compounded in her shroud, the stitches holding the fabric of life together not incongruous but in harmony with the mysterious depths from which they stemmed. Ned could only think of this harmony, in the shrine of daybreak, forsaking heavens canopy. There shone the sun that saves face every morning to send him into the clouds, she was definitely better than page three and better than the mirror too, scattering like light. Honesty keen like hopes, strangers knew each other now as part of some grand design; the heat of the sun shining upon them like the arc of a wing on the wind.

The radiant splendour of dawn was tranquil but they stood and ambled as surely as tiredness would take them to the square where the busses congregated. They smelt the first bread of the morning and the wine shops began their deliveries of huge oak barrels. Ned picked up a couple of bottles for a small amount of Euros. Someone shouted, "Here comes my drunken ship" as the bus arrived. Just as the joy of the morning had rubbed off on them they found themselves over a marshy river and the bus stopped at the road to the campsite. A desolate spot the only sign pointing to the beach; so they deliberated, agreeing to head in the opposite direction. Ned wanted to say something about not betraying her trust but as soon as they were at the gate he refrained. As the rose-beetle man approached them from inside Ned mumbled, "You're a tender soul" and left it at that.

The man was just as Ian had described him. The rose-beetle man was so called because he had small oval shaped rose-beetles hanging from his hand on pieces of string. His face was pointed with large slanting, brown eyes, which had a vacant, look about them. He was short and slimly built. He wore a green hat that had been faded by the sun, stained with wine and cigarette burns. In the floppy band round the hat there was an assortment of different birds' feathers as well as the wing of a kingfisher and the claw of a hawk. Around his neck a scarf made of blue satin hung tucked into his shirt. His shirt was frayed, worn and grey with sweat. His coat was festooned with patches; on the white patch were decorated rosebuds. The pockets were bulging with combs, little highly coloured pictures of the saints, olivewood carvings of snakes and dogs, cheap mirrors and a handkerchief. In one hand he carried a lit pipe, which he would sporadically puff upon as he spoke. He greeted them and took a noticeable self-depreciating attitude to Sian, such was his manner. He said that Ian had spent long nights talking. They entered to a swathe of bright green and flower-dispersed meadows of such wildness, dotted here and there by pregnant looking almond trees, that it was lushly breathtaking.

"Men eh…we'll tell you how to live then we'll take away the reason and we'll wonder why we wonder why you're not the way that we were…" After that he got confusing in broken English but soon enough he got down to formalities and as Sian sat on the firm ground Ned stood picking hungrily at the almonds. Curiously she did not go to Ian's room but hastily wrote a note telling him to meet her at the cathedral at two o'clock that day. Could Ned take this nonchalance as a small sign of coldness between them? Ian soon awoke, and as he left for work stopped in on her cabin. By this time however Ned was in his tent musing upon the day ahead and the night that had been. It was not too hot and he soon fell asleep, dreaming of being with her in a baroque castle like Percy and Mary Shelley.

It was two o'clock, the hands in perfect representation and the shadowy, narrow streets were cool and hemmed in from all sides. The living quarters, like the commercial districts breathed life into the area and they noticed an increase in people as they reached the luxuriousness of the cathedral piazza. The time continuum of intrigue and emotion had stood still here in the airy depths of the city where memories lay like catholic guilt in the hands of lovers who paraded the square. Shielded by umbrellas they sat down at a café illustrating previous patterns of a relaxed life, which enriched them like the coffee they sipped. As English people, Ned thought, that they had lived on feeling, not thoughts and sensation, which at a certain level leaves the primitive spirit more peaceful. Neither were particularly religious but they were confronted with the conditions to cultivate ideas of heaven's exist, within the boundaries of belief. They were aware that will to thought to belief and back again was the Christian message, not science and magick. To a catholic the spirit dwells in their thoughts of awareness and this led to a better-organized idea centre but a dumber sense of doubt. The cathedral was a hallowed ground, which called from ages not present to filter their awareness. They agreed that faith surrounded them like an affirmation of life but emotions must have a stop. Without harming their English expressions their ideas, opinions, mobility, deference, achievements, qualities, beliefs, commitments, goals and responses were conditioned by the sobriety of the square with a glowing resonance. The sun threw shadows on the stone and time asked where they had been. In the arms of another, tolled the bells as Ian strolled into view, emerging from the crowds like an Italian, full of attitude and swagger.

Ned pushed his shoulders forward as if they were the corners of a book he was trying to close and sat in mournful silence as the two greeted each other demonstratively. Ian sounded as he looked, with smart comments and well-phrased arguments. He was half Italian, handsome and not slight in stature. His suit pervaded an air of authority and his manner in ordering a coffee was just as brash. Ned had a flashback to running through dimly lit streets.

"First class that you got her here." He said with a vitriolic smile. Ned lifted his coffee and pretended to be pre-occupied with the flight. She told him of the beautiful mountains and drifting over the sea for hours. He told him of the sunrise and the confidence he had in the rickety old aircraft. It appeared that much remained unspoken in their relationship and he knew of her love for mystery but also of security. There was a false security in their passion which only Italian men can get away with, which was also where the mystery lay. Too unsure to be true, the rueful nature of his love for Sian was all he had compared to their passionate bravado.

"She's a girl in a million and I'm a millionaire," He laughed

"Business is treating you well then" interjected Ned before they had a chance to cuddle.

"Well I've got everything I want" and he gazed at Sian "now- as you've been in bed all day I had to leave you. I can't afford to be lazy"

"Bed is the poor mans opera," quipped Ned. Sian looked at him with full attention. Her boyfriend replied hesitantly

"And I must take you to the opera, Sian". She did not show the flower of her character to him. Their style was different as they talked. He found himself guarding the passions he felt, in case Ian took the Mickey out of them but anyway he was quite an amusing fellow and he did not ask for openness. A false friendliness ensued, the uneasy swiftness of their conversation pushing Ned's resentment to the fore until he made his excuses. Ian said that he had to be going back to work soon anyway and that he should stick around.

"I'll see you back at the rose-beetle campsite" Ian said after a while, and with a flourish of his napkin he was gone, leaving Sian visibly overwrought at the briefness of their encounter.

"Still" she mused, "the afternoon is in front of us and we should at least visit the catacombs before evening". After a last look around the square they departed, walking the way from the island to the old Byzantine church where the dead lay. The dead of a thousand years of Syracuse's finest. The streets were festooned with markets and clothes shops, the remnants of which were worn by the street vendors who looked smart although they only sold oranges. It was important for the citizens to look the part, even in death.

The steps leading down to the vault led like fish up and down, and the coldness of the hall greeted them like stepping into water. The crypt, an old Greek reservoir was huge and vaulted by stone arches. The frescos were faded and of Byzantine to Norman decoration but this was not what struck the two friends as they cherished the familiar correction-time game: these were the tombs of the dead. The bodies were all around, shrunken, limp and lifeless and stared down at the ground or heavens with mournful eyes in their dull, dark sockets. Ned didn't move but stared at the carcasses hanging from the walls like some unreal metamorphosis, the colour of moths. Their clothes were antiquated, faded but obviously their Sunday best; women robed in long, flowing grey dresses, men trussed up in dark, velvet suits. They looked like silence, as solace brought back the years. Many still clung to their youth as children, with wispy black hair flowing from sunken skulls. Their expressions were all different, though all the same- awestruck, as if caught in dreams. Teeth shone white from their ghastly form. The halls stretched as far as the eye could see, stretched in every direction. Sporadically there were ornate altars, temples to unknown saints lit up by the lights of a modern age. They walked among the passageways with solemnity, scattered here and there by grotesque conversation and dismay.

They soon became separated from the group and as Sian ran her hands along the wooden sarcophagus like the grains were strings, Ned stopped at an alter and read the inscription my eyes are those of a full life, a life you've never seen until you open my grave. As he read, he heard a piercing scream and followed its direction. A woman lay on the hard floor the eyes gauged out from her sockets; the freshness of the body struck deep contrast with the stretched, moth-eaten bodies around her and they were reaching out for the spilt blood. Ned arose in horror and returned to where he had left Sian. The bodies were swaggering towards her, and there, like a zombie, crouched a man dressed in a black cloak, his hands outstretched and pressing on her temples, thumbs over her beautiful brown eyes. Was this the certainty of chance? Ned felt a feeling surge up inside him and wrenched a skull from its owner. He thrust it at the man's head but it cracked and shattered upon his shoulders, leaving only dust upon his cloak.

The man turned and Ned and the man molded into one. He looked into his eyes and his eyes were eyes of his own. They struggled for which felt like an eternity, Ned finding courage and strength through his love for Sian that he had not expected. He was however overpowered and he collapsed helpless. When he revived he stepped disorientated to where Sian lay but as he did so a crowd descended upon him not free from rat nor mask. In his mind it was as though he had never escaped into the churchyard that night and he was still amongst the crowd on Serpentine road. However it was him whom they grabbed for the cloaked man, who despite his stature and strength had vanished. Beside him on the floor lay a document signed Jeremy Handlebars. As they searched the scene of the fight they produced two thick phials. Gleaming, as if caught in emotion were eight eyes.

Chapter 7 The Void

As the man was led away, he turned to Sian who was propped up against the wall. Her piercing eyes shone in disbelief and he could think nothing of his plight just the consternation he had seen in her. At the police station a message had been sent to England that they had found the eye trophy killer. The detective was suspicious. It was proved that Ned was in the docks when Rita Caprita was killed. "That's the most important piece of evidence we have yet," said the white rabbit as the synchronous labyrinth of chance carried on the same. The case was prepared with possessed ferocity to implicate Ned, and what could be called fabrication, by the detective codenamed the white rabbit. Ned went straight to an insane asylum due to his past history and the circumstantial motive of various strands of evidence in his rather confused diary and, of course, the eye of the surrogate sister. Claybury was a Victorian asylum when one man to each prison cell was a Victorian value.

To begin with Ned had a clear view of the doctor fraternity. Doctors have made the mysterious aspect of madness disappear; where people were once seen to be supernatural it is just another aspect of their illness. Another invented disease. The power has been taken by the doctors whom hold themselves to be shaman. Luckily enough as Ned had found out previously some of them are. They are made for life. We are mad for life. How many times must it be explained before the medical institution is taken from its pedestal? As for the drugs they peddled. Well they were only dangerous long term for they changed your reality not your behavior. Their pseudo-science changed the conditions.

As for his loss of freedom he soon adjusted. Freedom brings responsibilities after all. These were conditions of his incarceration, but his personality stayed the same. The trouble with the chemical world he inhabited was the four-seasons-in-one-day syndrome from your window bar. Addiction, cure, withdrawal and dependency became the seasonal routine. He missed nature and with that came the episodes of depression after a while. Just because you're paranoid doesn't mean that they're not out to get you. His favorite was the truth trip, which he had unfortunately when an old friend from university visited. He swung between trying not to make him angry, swearing blindly that he was the most interesting person he had ever met, and resenting him. He knew himself to be innocent, he thought as he sat in a drug-induced stupor while his friend in his wisdom sat with him, fearing that he was ultimately insane, as they really had always known. Needless to say he went for the seafood option. Seafood he knew invariably if mixed with the right amount of drugs produced all the signs of drunkenness.

Then there were the religious overtones. One nurse was famous on the ward for being a priest. He wasn't but continued to take confession from the prettier of the girls. The other nurses were just as bad, walking around in black, grinning and flustering. I mean Nazis go around thinking they are better than everyone else, wear black and are self-righteous. Nurses well. One inmate was convinced that the trophy killer was the devil. He announced one day squinting out of one eye as he talked: "It was not the hands of a man but a harvest, which tempted the innocent of a generation. The devil produces with malice and wonder a lavish deceit into every man's core. The unremitting evil he enacts is a terrible temptation. Everyone wants the same thing don't they? The devil does too. He just wants to corrupt the innocent, regale honesty, defile truth, and make everything under his control. That is what everyone wants isn't it? This is how he torments you and pulls us down to the depths." He also believed that *his* old man was the devil but it was nice to feel that someone was on your side.

The best time was when a disreputable but lovable character visited Ned and insisted upon being let in himself, drunk and scowling. His dog would not let any of the goon squad near him to escort him off the premises. He just sat there; scowling menacing and howling telling everyone he was mad. Light relief Ned thought. The doctors questioning was a trial but soon Ned learnt to cope. It always began the same when Robach entered the room. Ned would be silent and he would try to wheedle an insanity out of him: "There is a strand of truth in every opportunity one takes. Knowledge can be a fine thing but often, by definition, the kindling of experience can destroy innocence. Or you could do away with innocence?" Ned was resilient that way. Robach was not subtle. He was a persistent psychiatrist, and not overly gifted but had a good reputation down the social for being a joker. He was not, however, very balanced when it came to detective work. He couldn't see the wood for the trees. Hence he had not risen as quickly as ambition asked of him.

Respite did occur in the form of sport, art and music therapy that he enjoyed, but the real joy was the maddest of the women who would go from really mad to completely lucid. When mad she would stand behind your chair brushing your hair and singing sweetly. When well she would completely ignore you. It reminded Ned of Sian. Sian was confused; it was not that she thought he was guilty; it was just that she did not know who had attacked her. Something that the white rabbit used to implicate Ned. But Ned had been pissed on from a large height. One night he contemplated suicide and held the knife in his hands. The world will be wonderful they say but from whose perspective? The last fantastic book took one look at a world where justice no longer took hold, screwed up its eyes and jumped on, up, into the darkness.

He saw Sian only once. He thought that she got perverse pleasure from it, though in reality she hated every moment. She rose to the occasion and told Ned of her journey on the tube. You never could really tell if she was serious or not: *"Incredible! fascinating! We journeyed this morning on the void train. Whether it was doomed, I will never know. I thought at first it was a normal morning, I woke up one minute before my alarm, my dad burst in half a minute before and I turned it off 10 seconds before it was due. The blasted thing does annoy me on the best of days and if it does finally have its say, I am welcomed into that world by a trumpet fanfare directly into my left ear, most unbalanced- this noise often played by the best trumpeter, can surely not receive the appreciation that is truly due to it. So I shot from bed, got ready, had breakfast and went on my way. The bus was just pulling away and luckily pulled in my direction, so barely stopping, we seemed to merge together and journeyed toward Hainault station.*

On the platform, I received a prod, quite harsh, on the shoulder and it was an acquaintance from school. I had seen her on occasion since then so I wasn't that shocked but was trying to think of other people from school I had seen since I last saw her. I decided to give in. I couldn't be bothered and it was obvious to me that she felt likewise as when we boarded, she shoved her head into her EVA magazine and huddled around her bag adorned with white cat hair (or was this the pattern).

I briefly looked at the others rushing into my carriage. Almost sucked into their chairs, they quickly opened their other worlds and were gone. Some were most annoyed when their chairs were taken and knew from this that they were in for a bad day. The void train drew away from the station and everybody nestled to the comforting racket. The first time I was certain of this world was at Gants Hill. A Spanish dancer got onto the train. He was a man of about fifty with grey hair and blue eyes. With one arm raised back and high above his head and holding a vertically striped plastic guitar around his neck, he gallivanted through the carriage, quite unnecessarily, to the next. There he stopped to entertain the crowd.

Then I noticed that sitting opposite to myself, slightly to the right was Ruth (and I know this from a tacky dress-ring she wore on her left hand). She looked at me intensely for just a split second and poised her claws. Her nails were the longest I have ever seen but perfectly kept and painted deep maroon, almost black. Ruth was proud of her hands, each finger had a ring of some sort and one was a diamond butterfly. She clutched the old fashioned telephone on her lap tightly but not too tight to obscure her nails. She had nothing to read; nothing to do but stare and clutch and wait.

The non-characters by now were hoarding onto the void train, each opening their little worlds to block that one. I looked along to where Ruth sat and there was a Vicar in his own little world – a modest Bible. He was in his mid-forties; his hair was blonde-grey and thin and surrounded his head like a shining halo. His face was long and his beak nose pointed in the direction of the psalm he read.

The void train passed Leytonstone – It was bleak there. The roofs were in tatters and the pigeons perched like Kings proud of their castles. One shrieked a sharp and disturbing tone towards the void train as it pulled away from the station and continued to be heard for the rest of my journey. Although more distant, it seemed more intense and frightening and my heart began to beat faster. I decided that I would get off at the next stop as these characters were beginning to threaten me.

A woman in the appropriate attire tiptoed through the carriage with her cake trolley tempting people with her wares. The non-character were quite amused by this and obliged to taste the offering.

The trolley was a glass case and inside mounted on a velvet plinth was the biggest and most delicious looking chocolate digestive biscuit. Their eyes were full of greed and each non-character was handed a portion of this delight, which they ate in haste. The anxiety was urging me to stay part of this void journey. I looked into the glass next to where I was sat (I always choose to sit in the corner so I can lean and so I only have to bear the warmth of one non-character next to me). Someone with a black material jacket was leaning the other side of the glass patrician and I could then obtain a discrete but quite accurate view of other characters. And there behind his Times paper stood Jack Nicholson himself! I could hardly breath at the menacing sight and could not peel my eyes away from the jacket he was in. I frantically looked to where he was really standing and there; he was just an innocent looking ginger-haired man with a fair complexion. His colouring had altered my perception only through the black jacket he stirred the most abusive fright.

We passed the Cemetery where one of Jack the Rippers' wives were buried and Ruth took a glance at Jack N. My whole body shuddered; I could no longer control this scene. The doors opened at Leyton and on walked the Ripper himself in a black and white small-checked coat, roughly shaven and ready for work. It dawned on me that everyone was preoccupied but Ruth and Himself and he looked so bloody normal, such a city gent. How dare he use such a disguise! I continued to hear the pigeons shriek amongst the roar of laughter coming from the consecutive carriage. The non-characters mesmerized by the Spanish scene – other non-characters from my carriage had now joined them to recommend the digestive delight. The trolley maid was summoned to that carriage and another biscuit was lifted from the case – a cheer ripped through all carriages. Like starved animals, they rampantly feasted until they were full. Then, they danced furiously on what was left, pulping it down to crumbs, rubbing themselves with it and dissolving their skin. In ecstasy they danced, shear delight, screams of pleasure. Other non-characters joined and the orgy of sex, noise and death began until – on approaching Stratford, the huge monster pie had eaten itself.

Stratford was still, with the exception of the pigeon's bionic cry. Jack R stood unashamed in the corner and moved his hand toward his coat pocked to produce a mobile phone. Ruth flinched and held tighter to hers. They were a conspiracy! I was sure now and was near to madness and growing weak. I could envisage no way out.

I turned my attention to my friend who was still busily reading her magazine, how could she so easily ignore the massacre that had just occurred in the next carriage? How could she ignore her carriage that housed the two most evil jacks and Ruth? I began to panic. On the back of her magazine was the man from UNCLE – he tilted his cap and waved at me.

At Bethnal Green stepped another of our absurd visitors. She was wearing a rust coloured coat with big brown lines in check. My eyes followed up from her coat to her face and to my horror, her eyes had been painted by the devil. Thick black liner surrounded them and had been drawn outwards toward her temples. I wasn't clear who she was but she certainly belonged to someone here.

Ruth got off at Liverpool Street, Jack N and R had already gone. This woman had also vanished from sight, yes – they were a trio of some sort as I had suspected. No! There she was, sat in Ruth's seat. Her hands were in view now, they were green and furry and slimy – she was a reptile. I looked at the vicar who had aged about 30 years whilst he had sat there and the pigeons continued to cry. A non-character brought an offering from Bank but it was accepted by no one so she ate it herself in disgust.

I got off of the void train at St Paul's at 8.25 on a fine autumn day, along with the non-characters that were left and we ascended toward the light. We left behind such a passionate scene of animals and weirdom quite beyond belief. Who would enter the void train next? We will never know" © Lorraine Bearryman. She had begun work in London. Ned however was vehement to prove to her his innocence. He began

"It is curious that the eye trophy killer didn't realize the motivation of his crime. Finding a motive is like the disposal of a shroud", he said; "the relief and texture of every lovers dream is like the revealing of a bust of Homer being watched by Aristotle, being painted by Rembrandt. Compulsion is the key, compulsion. The man must be obsessed. The obsession spawns until it takes on a mythical shroud. Its colour is fervor; rich and deeply sumptuous and like Caesar's shroud, the colour consists of time's stock- serial killers consistently produce remarkably similar patterns as the previous crimes. It is like a set of keys; yearnings latched onto by evil. The permanence in change, the lock itself perhaps, is the flow of time entombed by the past. It unalterably determines our journeys in the present. The killer was me but it wasn't me." He had confused her fully and she broke down in tears and he was led away. That was when Ned planned his escape.

Out of the body of depression a plan emerged. He had an innate fascination with the spiral tree. It seemed to draw him to it. He planned the escape with military precision. He stole the key to the consultancy room; made a rope with sheets he saved from the laundry and made a note of when the laundry van came each morning. The night of his escape he laced the dogs dinner with tranquillisers and sat in his bed waiting. He got a friend to piss on the floor and while the nurse was dealing with that, he slipped into the corridor. He fished the bunch of keys from a nurse's belt in the confusion and opened the dormitory door. He then opened the consultancy door and wriggled through the open window. He crouched low as the rope took his weight and jumped to the ground. He ran to a bush. Sure enough the guard dog was dozy and disorientated so did not notice him. As the laundry van pulled up he slipped through the fence gateway. His freedom was assured as he neared the outer perimeter for his friend, the scowling character had cut the fence. He walked into the street and was once more normal, sane, free. If of course that was what the early morning void was.

He amused himself upon his walk by imagining what life would be like without money, as in the dark ages when the Romans left. When the fountain of the void stopped no one knew, maybe last Wednesday. As it used to spew forth the pennies the nuns sat around waiting for the penny to drop and accepted them gleefully as the real change from the duties they were resigned to. The alters of the cash machines stood, like lustful fountains, continually sending forth credits to the leaders of the nuns. A few even took their stares away from the road but as soon as they had bathed their brittle hands in money they soon returned to the pointless staring and absorbed looks at anyone who dared to enter their part of the void. After all conversation was saved for those you knew, and it was best to get the point away as efficiently as possible. I tried to be subtle about the day I left behind but soon returned to gibberish about a trainer and its owner.

A couple had stood on the verge of lust, for as he collected denominations of currency from the fountain he exclaimed "loaded!" and that was enough to calm the resentment she held for their meaningless existence. What do you get for being in love anyway? she thought, but now the cash machine, the fountain of all monies, refused to grant to the nuns. Suddenly wistful of its role, over the next couple of weeks the money, which had always flowed to form puddles on the ground, dried up: the couple broke up as he was no longer a man, the only currency being the message that each and every one handed out as advice. Ned picked up a piece of paper from the road. In the desert we are all blind. It said.

Ned felt stranger than ever as he entered the void. It felt as though the work-crowds had fixed him with a steadfast gaze, which could see right through him like a rabbit caught in the open from up high. He felt overshadowed and had to run the gauntlet of eyes that made him feel frail and shallow, the shallowness of equity with them touched his soul. He passed the plastic shops with their mannequins staring like the people who passed him by into the void. People were meant to be excited by the plastic world these mannequins created. To buy the clothes, the jewelry, the widescreen TVs- plastic temptation presented by the void.. Ned's strand of insanity was to blame himself and twist the rag in further.

Just walking around in a circle of romantic self-destruction- so superficial- how utterly plain and unoriginal! He admired the deviants, thank god for their originality. And nature- my word she's in control. Human beings I cry- so superior? With our beautiful concrete jungles and clothes, and cake from the seed, and pets from the field and strut it dear on the catwalk and shoot your silver precious bullet and slice down trees with your metal smog carriage and burn holes in the sky with your air fresheners. His paper-cut wounds were slight yet peoples pockets throbbed with the misery of sullen wallets as a non-character wandered gormlessly by with his bag of provisions. He peered onwards down his narrow corridor, his choice of doorways very limited. How insignificant the vessels of humankind only for their blood to be sucked by their screaming vermin- "Sorry the TV broke because my little darling put her dummy through the screen" he heard from a shop front in the high street.

It was not that he was scared but he wanted the hand that rocked the cradle. He wanted to speak to his father. He wanted that security he had never had. He wanted the answer all the other boys had been given. He wanted Sian. He wanted to be set free. He wanted to belong. The labyrinth of his mind turned to the reality that he had grown susceptible in the void so that he craved the airy depths of the asylum. Just because you have the perception of abstract ideals there's no need to turn the world into a circling carrion-filled society. We start off, full of ideals of equality and romance when what women really need is someone to take decisions from them, a lover who will take over. Then there's the sense that a man needs a maid- someone to hand him his tie in the morning and however hard you try its impossible to get away from those stereotypes. The sickening reliance on the pretence of capitalism follows. If the hen wants to go into the wolf's mind does she have to enter the wolf's den? He could see quite clearly the exclusiveness of their wares but to cope one had to rage against it. It was a dangerous place for the innocent to be. They fuck you up so they can fuck you up. The vicious nature of those things parted by the non-world is painted concrete grey. Just as it is the mark of an ecologist not to sweep the plain truths of a youth's mind under the carpet, so society should be a means to an end. It should rally against politicians whose misused promises never took responsibility. We should instill a *green* tradition to fill the gaps between the shibboleths we chase. But not solely to the mentally ill are events desolation characterized by loyalty to the bourgeois mentality. The pulp of malevolent culture avaricely presented by modern technology, at the ad-mans' expertise is the only self-discovery. He mustered his resentment. He had

found the hand that cradled the rock and the
labyrinth awaited him.

Chapter 8 Labyrinthine

Ned sat as he had sat many times before, on the hill in the outskirts of the forest overlooking progress; the mediocre buildings stretched before him not planned
but a monstrous sprawl with no sign of diminishing or giving up the ghost in any direction. All through the circling years the train of progress had crept, eating into the
countryside until it met the impenetrable barrier of an ancient forest whose roots stood firm against encroachment, defending the earth like a large foraging army, which lived in the trees who pushed memories into sprigs of salt. He was drawn towards the spiral tree. Ned sat in a circle of romantic self-destruction and wrote

Love over regret
Like a lake rippling
With suffocating rain
Fell upon your windows
And shone ghostly
Of sorrow and pain
Love over regret

As he did so he absentmindedly dug hollows in the earth with his heels. His attention was taken by a hollow sound. He thought it the remains of roots over perhaps a rabbit warren but no; it was an area six foot by six foot square. Strange he thought. Strange that nothing grew here.

He began to rummage through the leaves and thin layers of mulch, which covered it, not expecting to find anything in particular. There it was, a wooden pallet shaped square at his feet. As the hustlers hustled in the city below he opened it and crept inside holding up his lighter to see into the blackness. Inside was silence, musty and colluded with the spiders that had been the only visitors there for perhaps a millennium. He found a candle and lit it. Suddenly as though a magic spell had been caste, the room was visible, a small chamber with a plethora of macabre and strange but wonderful objects. What caught his attention firstly were the shelves of books all bound in dark but almost transparent leather.

He saw the sorcerer within the cloak had withered like his dress, and had no brightness but the brightness of his sunken eyes. He was covered by a thinly hanging shroud the colour of which, however designed, was the damp, coarse colour of the walls, muddy purple. Now the skeleton seemed to have dark eyes that moved and looked at him. He should have cried out, if he could.

An axis had turned to present Ned with a view from beyond the mists of time and space. The hid-hole of an ancient shaman whose story had been long forgotten. He almost expected the walls to come tumbling in but what he had discovered lay asleep until this day and had now been awoken by the march of time. He made the chamber into his hideout and concealed from the outside world, he devoured the books of the warlock.

He had written to Sian the day before his escape and had told her that if she trusted him at all she should meet him by the spiral tree on this date. So it was that she decided to take the chance and meet a fugitive in Epping Forest. Epping forest had been an ancient Iron Age fortress; the people of ages past had lived and breathed where he stood for thousands of years while the forest stood steadfast through all religious persuasion. The druids had respect for the seasons and no fear of death. They believed in the immortality of the soul. The soul moved into another body and as it grew and changed, the season's mysteries unfolded. Metempsychosis.

He was at the Iron Age camp in the woods and he likened to the ripeness in the land. He was waiting as he had waited a hundred times before, but since last month waiting was not the same. This was his last chance to bring Sian round. He collected firewood and soon the fire caste flickering shadows on the ground and over the element of darkness. He noticed the spiral tree and the firm shadow it cast in contrast to the dancing shadows around him. The fire caught him in a spell and seemed to speak to him: "I....", Ned jumped from his muse "...I shall conceal; the blame- Come, come to me. I have seen you at your worst; the spiteful, bitter sore will disappear if only you draw near. I....", Ned cast his eyes hither "....I will bring you jewels in my arms. Sink, sink into me. I read you like a book, adventures, pictures galore will come alive if only we contrive. I....." Ned stretched out his arm. "I will devour your dreams Glow, glow with me. I will throw you pearls of the past, the sacred core will sooth if only you move into the fire. I....", Ned reached into the flames "...I will raise you like a phoenix- Rise, rise with me. I will glorify you in my arms, the life you bore will last if only you are caste....The sinister fire in the body of waiting indulged his fatalism and he only just heard footsteps approaching. Enter the scene the hourglass figure.

Ned was almost compelled to throw the book he was holding into the fire, but drew back from his indulgence. "You know you were saying about travelling- getting there before you started. Well I think I, or should I say this book has cracked it. Time travel I mean. Its called *Labyrinthine.*" They both looked at the green covered collection of pages in his hand. "Its in old English but I think I've worked it out. Central to its magic is that cosmic forces betray the past through the perihelion; a measure of how we perceive the world. I found it in the hand of a skeleton in his chamber in the forest and I've kept silent till now, too afraid of what people might say. This is kind of about me; this is kind of about you. It is most definitely about my guilt." They talked excitedly and fast for an hour or so, and though she thought he really was mad she succumbed and poured over the book as one might an heirloom or picture album.

Do we travel through time by thinking of situations long since gone, or is it the thing that dreams are made of? The labyrinth was contained within our gene-pool, a destiny that will be played out irrespective of our choices in life. Perceived through the perihelion, knowledge persisted throughout, waiting to be revealed by experience. One knew everything one needs to know and life was its discovery. The labyrinth was a chain of events over time and though the initial conditions may be changed, trying was the meaning of life; belief the point. The Labyrinthine concluded that individuals could not control the outcome of destiny. Fundamentals had repercussions throughout time and these fundamentals could not change. The labyrinth was a tapestry whose detail could be changed but whose patterns remained the same. One had the possibility of opening a new door but, as long as one closed it behind them, the perception would be the same. Time travel was a function of perception and this was what controlled time.

Chapter 9 Chariot of Fire

"I must say an incantation to awake the majesty of Boudicca," Sian held the dog-eared papers in her hand as she spoke. "We are lost souls, Boudicca, angel of soul, the puzzles which I called my fear so hopeful that it may explain my introspective core. I see my ruin as the wet ground. Wherever you go I will follow". A mistress of illusion and caution she sat on the ground and looked out upon the torn grace of the spiralled tree. Sian blinked. She was somehow lost for years like a ladder in the snow, until she grasped the meaning of the tall edifices and the charmed heather as common ground with the ancestors. She continued; "Innocence and honesty are notions around my wrists and my heart reminisces to disclose your heart, which like the moon, the remains of your golden chariot, wells from the fire." Sian looked at the tree. There on its bark were two names Ned and Sian carved into it. "This is a good omen" said Sian, and then said forcefully "Wait". She bent down and carved a heart and arrow through between them. She spoke, stroking her embarrassment from her hair. "Good thoughts are like friendliness, they always say hello. Someday I'd be careful as each precious moment passed away. Queen of balance and touch, break the barred entrance of the bough, heaving in the mystical windswept air. I pluck a strand of my hair, consoling a journey through the silver berths, your portal of ages, my passion to save."

"According to the middle part of the book we pass through the portal to tread the labyrinth of our ancestors. It mentions about far reaching paradoxes. A traveller will go back in time and know our futures. That is one. That we might merge is another"

"Well are you ready" she said excitedly, used to stumbling on the unknown. "How else are we to find out if it is real or not?"

"OK, we have to carve on the foot of the tree what time we are to appear in. I looked it up that when Boudicca was here was in the autumn of AD 61."

"Go on then" she said, "where can we go but to despair if it isn't true?" She carved the date onto the tree and climbed hesitantly into the tree. She hung as if waiting for an important phone call and then swung her feet downward. She dropped what would have been the small drop through the spiral of the tree but a mist closed around her as she travelled labyrinthine. There was a rush of wind and a sickly smell with the stars shooting around her as if travelling though the cosmos or childbirth. They drifted for a few minutes and then with a bump she crashed to the ground. Thinking that it was nothing but a fall Sian turned to look at Ned - but it wasn't Ned at all.

She stood up. "I think I realize what love comes from," she interjected but it was not her voice at all. It was not even her language. Sian was aware of many lives' wisdom clearing in her head as if overtaking the thoughts she had been having. She was a collective of the lives that she had experienced compounded in this form. One thing was clear - life would never be the same again. Sian had in her hand a strand of her hair.

Ned was left in the forest alone, in his hand the book. As she jumped through the tree a mist descended and at first ghostlike she disappeared from view.

She looked slightly darker in her complexion but around the same age. The hair seemed to have an innate attraction to her. "You know the whole desire of the world is contained within its fragility". She was trying to come to terms with the situation. She felt strung out as if in a drug induced rush of foresight, both pain and pleasure. Physicality was less important to her but she could express the senses better and with an ever-increasing vitality. The truths of sorrow and pleasure in a calmness she had not felt before was the broad prosaic result.

There was a beat in the background and she was aware of being in the throng of a huge encampment, interspersed with fires and wagons but mostly people, lots of people all similarly and rudimentally dressed as she was. "You're a relic, you're just a fashion accessory," she concluded.

"I saw my metal in a flash of moonlight glinting from up high." Taken by his invincible form she looked at the man by her side and was aware of primitive lust in her. Her emotions however were to spurn the type of man that thrust attention on her but with a movement that would bruise tired lips he swung downward and kissed her.

"What's your name?" said Sian

"What's in a name? He turned. "The flame that warms something you can't conceal from the fire I give you in the dark. My name is fire" He was however the same as the roman generals who had tried to woo her and who had ultimately broken her resolve.

"I something you, somewhat me" she spoke.

Beside them, a little to the right sat the sage Amairgin, blue tattooed shank and beard of grey and from three cauldrons there came an almighty stench. The wizened old man spoke of the volary of the broth, established by diligence and inspiration and overturned by joy. He commanded the man to be seated for the stock of rebirth, whence each art is dispensed. He then turned and waved a wand over the steaming cauldron. To conjure the goodness of the blessed, Sian threw in her strand and it lit up the night with a brief flash and returned to the element of darkness. Amairgin lifted a ladle full of the broth as the folk around him lifted their bowls. He went to the darkest corner first and ladled the bowl; a figure that emerged into the firelight as a vision of the old ways was a woman whose fiery fierceness in her face would rein a horse, or issue limbs from smoky mouths, or makes flee enemies to be dissolved in elements. Her eyes gleamed in the firmament. It was the Celtic queen Boudicca, the phantom phoenix from the flames and spear, which glistens through the air writhing as once her daughters did under the swathes of roman heads now over her shoulder.

"To rid this Caesars grip, in the forest awnings of red and yellowing leaves to the land of brooks- lest the forests turn to plains and the plains to forests. *They shall be decoyed to their doom at Colchester. We British are used to women commanders in war. I am fighting as an ordinary person for my lost freedom, my bruised body and my outraged daughters. The gods will give us the vengeance we deserve! The Roman division that dared to fight is annihilated. The others cower in their camps. They will never face even the din and roar of all our thousands, much less the shock of our onslaught. Look and see how many of you are fighting- and what you are fighting for- and why! Then you will win this battle, or perish.* We will never submit to the roman yolk. For rebirth of the slain - a toast! My anguish turns in my soul but sorrow I do not feel. Their deaths were not in vain. All for glory"

Nor science, nor magic, nor imagination, nor Halloween festivities could console her. She had decided to find the legions and give up the fruits of their labours, the one thing she could rely upon, the harvest. Sian was in the pale moonlight alone, tramping through the red and yellowing crushed leaves under her sadness which she could not impress anyone with, trying to contact mother earth to pay her dues, to relinquish her soul and pride she had in her relationship. She could not consider any man in this life as a lover. Was this a paradox? She felt like the waning moon, empty as though her soul was a small blurred thing she held in his hand ready to throw into the dark waters of the lake, the entrance to the afterworld, barred to all but the warrior.

She hadn't wanted to fight but the truth has a habit of coming home and it was as though she had a primeval urge to spill blood. As she delved between trees she heard something only heard late at night. The popping and clicking of a fire. She approached and as she did her mother, Boudicca, shimmering in the moonlight and shadows flickering like the dance of a sword lit her view, blessings stretched over her lines of grey muslin. She steadied her nerve and she gave her sadness and she in turn showed her cowardice in love's indulgence. She felt guilty. She jangled a bunch of keys provocatively.

"This is the key to my heart," she said. "This is the key to my sexuality," she said. "This is the key to my soul." As she spoke she ushered Sian to the side where three doors stood.

" I do not deserve your heart" she said " for I have a true heart and live forever in its midst. The union of sex is enticing and is my desire, but it is too fleeting and its fire would burn my memory to cinders. I choose your soul for it is the door to mother earth whose forgiveness I have to endure for taking a vulnerable soul and dashing it upon the rocks in battle."

She turned the key in the heavy door and it opened gently. As though she had vanquished a feeling, serenity and peace engulfed her contradicting with the approach of a storm, bringing the world gusting towards her containing letters, which she never meant to send. In front of her but all around was a huge space, dark but filled with a million lights.

"What you see is what you want," said a strange hallowed voice. As she looked into mystery it was a childhood scene, the hustled adulation of a crowd, the peace of a country village, the dismay of missing someone; but overriding it all, a feeling of fulfilment in a moment of truth until she was floating on hope and fear. She felt at one with her surroundings but part of it and emanating from herself and the feeling of another, closer than fiction, was the mystery of cherished moments exploding from pinnacles of light. The sense of female energy engulfed her and she felt like being caressed by a hundred warming hands massaging the pressures, limits and spiritual wants she harboured. Her achievements were beauty, and beauty knowledge, so that all creation was suddenly known to her and she felt Gods loneliness until sensation returned to her and she was in the pale moonlight by the fire. In her hand was a ring of stone, which captured the universe like the summer loving she had known as a teenager; she knew that the present was forever and that the battle was rife.

Needless to say Boudicca addressed her troops before the steadfast roman legions with triumphant words along the Essex Way: *Though a woman my resolution is fixed, the men if they please may survive with infamy and live in bondage, on this spot we must either conquer or die with glory: there is no alternative.*

The Celts rushed into the affray but had to run uphill. Javelins decimated them and although they looked to the batteries of spears the Romans closed ranks behind shields and repelled them. The roman general rallied his troops calling the Celts disorganized rabble. They advanced with a parry of javelins. The approaching firestorm buffeted the army, which was so closely packed that they could only see the sky and could not swing their swords for the crush. The stabbing advance of the determined highly organized Roman legions cut through the army in short stabbing formations. The Celts were braced but although Boudicca and her daughters rode into the lines they and their chariots made little headway and were cut down by arrows. The Celtic form of warrior ship was in the height of battle just a gesture. The braver of the men advanced and were cut down, the rest waited until they were boxed in between the wagons and advancing Romans. The Romans spared no one and as a javelin hurtled through the air Bodicca fell. 56 chariots broke the lines and surrounded her and her daughters. They brought back her body. Standing back from the scene of carnage, Sian took it upon herself to break the ranks and fight their way out towards London with the body.

Sian was tired and desolate. Their chance had dissolved and indeed been wrenched from their grasp. Initial ferocity had been returned with scorn. As the battle unfolded their hopes diminished. They were not the thunder, they were not the rain and the fiercest of their elements, the blood curdling calls had fallen on deaf ears. The relief was palpable as they joined the forest on the border of Essex and returned to the Loughton camp. They had to act quickly. The Romans were following up their rout by sending out advance parties of soldiers looking for the queen and their intelligence was excellent. Many of the Celts had turned to grass and disappeared. Their potential was the ears of corn, which fall to the ground unmolested to make next years harvest. Sian went up to her body- reality is a row of devious paths through which we find happiness: happiness is knowing you have stood up for what you believe in. She seemed to say from her wan pale lips. There was only a skeleton of the former glory and with these they went to a sacred site, a chamber on the clay summit of Baldwins Hill. They prepared for burning the body. Sian as one of her daughters lit the pyre of her chariot with solemnity.

"I don't want to undermine the tenure of your feelings in defeat but in life the degree you love, commit, realize, reason, recognize and live life to the full was the clear vision of what you required from people and places. You like they paid the highest sacrifice". Forty thousand Celts on the roman road perished through one last dance to rid this Caesars' grip over this land of brooks and manna. The body of such vigor lay as crumpled hopes, the sanguine colour of a pale and luminous moon. As her ringlets showed through the earthy midnight air her body was sent to chariots fire to rise and shine each new day. The spiral tree murmured and sprung into life.

The tree stood as the portal of the labyrinthine and after a period of mourning the corpses ashes were lowered into a secret chamber enclosing spells, which entombed time. The *labyrinthine* commanded that she return. However she knew that the sun had crossed her path forever. Evoking the spirits Sian stood by the spiral tree. It was still dark. She uttered an incantation and carved the date of her home time on the bark. A spark engulfed her and fizzled around her body like a Catherine wheel. She was in a deep dark forest and could make out the monoliths of trees. However there was the eye trophy killer dressed in a cloak there. She was one with him. She was the old man!

Chapter 10 Great Expectations

Let me sink into your madman's dream. With that Ned carved 1890 on the tree and climbed gingerly into the tree. Like waiting for a weekend his feelings were mixed. He saw his thoughts turn to the lost souls of heaven who walk on the ground and within a labyrinth of ancient memory his mind stretched and swung from the lives of his ancestors. Time played upon him. However before he could fully realize them, he was within the forest clearing listening to two lads laughing. Did he really belong to this world? His body was that of his great grandfather, he recognized from old motheared photographs, and he hollered out his name in the darkness. His two friends, Aldous and H. followed suit caught up in the ribaldry of a forest walk. They were on their way to pay homage to Dickens at The Olde Kings Head, Chigwell. They had a weekend of partying at Copped Hall where they had spent the morning communing with the sun and ivory statues in the great garden. All three dreamed of being authors.

They frolicked over the forest ground to the edges of cultivated land. Many fields and large houses looming across them but little sign of the clutter of modern living. Three silhouettes hastened from the brow of the hill. The river's fields stretched from bank to orchard to field with only a new station and a clutter of improvised buildings of Buckhurst Hill greeting them. However the whole of Albert, Queens and Victoria Roads were festooned with bunting and the trappings of a royal visit. For this was what the three were going to see. To lean out of the fifteenth century pub's window and watch Queen Victoria pass in her colonnade towards these isolated buildings they were passing.

They stopped by the riverbank to have a smoke and puffing from pipes they felt very grand. Neither of them had drunk ale before, only a little sherry on occasions, as they were only 17. There's was a trip to an inn and Aldous had booked the Dickens room for the occasion. The mood was light and bright, wonderful ideas flicked between them interspersed with gay songs of the era. Their favorite was about Jack the Ripper and they sang as they walked:

Creeps up, eyes shut, your bleedin' throat's cut
The ripper's gonna get you if you don't watch out

"You are no nearer catching me than you were three years ago". Shouted the boys in unison. They had an innate fascination with him as did most of London at the time. They approached Chigwell and Ned saw his old school in the distance; little had changed.

Pubs in those days were places for all of society: intelligencer, landed gentry, artisans, backroom boys, and the farming community all shared the same roof, if only for a few hours and there was a ribaldry which intoxicated all; mixing drinks, position and stories. They were uncommonly good places.

Evening trade was just getting started when they entered, dusted down their coats and customarily stared around the wooden beamed inn. Before they had much chance to get their bearings Aldous went up to the bar and challenged the barman to find them the best whiskies in the house and producing a denomination far larger than usual, took the initiative. Drinks in hand they had succeeded. The company was colorful and soon the open fire and the misted windows brought contentment like they had been there forever.

"That we should be here, enjoying the simple things in life, is very complex don't you think? Time is a simple scenario but look at all the intricate probability it took for us all to be here. The odds are alarming." Said William.

"Destiny is often simple, my dear fellow. We are meant to be together." Replied Aldous.

"Destiny is the most complex effect of mans' existence I would surmise", said H. "We have first to look at these two elements. Take music for instance. The musical process is both simple and complex but can lead to great simplicity or intricacy. Indeed there are simple building blocks- rhythm, melody and harmony, which build a complex structure but when the piece is finished it reverses itself. It is simple again."

"Metaphysically the creative process in itself means that something has to come from nothing, but for something to come from nothing, nothing has to be something in the first place."

"Sex is simple. You haven't had it. You're as white as a sheet, white as the virgin snow. Not so me. That's because I do what I want. You do what you ought. I learn from experience, you learn from what is taught." Retorted Aldous

"The taut white sheet that covers that girl's secret night I suppose." They laughed. Conversation flowed like this for the rest of the night but soon the clientele dispersed among whispers and hollow jollity.

"Where does the time go? I think the pumps are closed."

"Not to worry, I've a bottle of whisky and the night is young. Let us retire to our room and await the queen!", and with that Aldous ushered them upstairs.

The Dickens suite was sumptuous; the décor was hung up on that happiness thing, each piece of furniture chosen for its merit not its blending quality. They blended the whisky and sat in the old leather seats. William looked at the window, while H. looked down the crack in the floor wishing to catch a glimpse of the lady downstairs through half-drunk eyelids. "That don't mean a thing if you can't sing..." The clarity of the situation felt like a dream but the historian in him was fascinated by the original prints of the great man himself. Who could tell that he was sitting with the greatest literary geniuses of the 20th century?

"We are in great company," said William examining a manuscript on the wall

"His mum told him a trip was a fall, when one is quite obviously not the other," Aldous said as H. fell over.

"Excuse me" said H. The three chatted excitedly for a while but the drunkenness got the better of them. This drunken night they concluded that thought was the slave of life!

"....The 19th century panders to the first in an all-or-nothing philosophy. That mind is nothing but a tool for making tools controlled by reflexes of nature or nurture's pressures. Our expressions are..."

"Our expressions are to affirm reality upon thought, sullied by earthly stain. I transpose instead of feel, and to summon all before you in your mind is to live in an ivory tower", said William.

"Thought is only our construction of time, a convention", replied H. "I would not lie in an ivory tower with orthodoxy. Lying in state like the old methods of systematic thinking, the queer absurdities of the Aristotelian logic, mystical numbers, and the blackness of the unthinkable. Expression is a perception, the fancies that made all ancient peoples speak of their gods only by circumlocutions, that made savages pine away and die because they had been photographed, or an Elizabethan farmer turn back from a day's expedition because he had met three crows"

"All quite true but if it were true then that would be the proof that it were false." Added Aldous. Inebriated they fell asleep.

The prosperous and good of Essex, and then again the poor and unworthy lined the streets from the villages of Ilford to the country retreats of Chigwell. The level of noise broke the pallid daylight in the room. William woke with a start and roused the others. They ordered cooked breakfast from downstairs and hung the large lead paned windows wide just as the queens carriage passed by heralded by the queens life guards, looking like penguins on an arctic trail. The large black frosted windowed carriage sped past with horses pulling in graceful procession and sinews of power. The illusive ice-queen was probably as frail inside as the monarch's idea of Utopia.

"So that's the empress of India is it" said H.

"That's providence for you I suppose" moaned Aldous. It was, needless to say, a bit of an anticlimax but William soon roused their spirits by suggesting that they walk to the spiral tree, which he busily explained during their ample breakfast, was the key to the book he presented to them as they were eating: The *Labyrinthine.* Aldous stood back and exclaimed sarcastically that he didn't believe in magic since he had seen the conjurer's trick box, but H. was far more taken by the idea and began to talk excitedly of a project he had been working on about the scientific exploration of the future.

"This could be it!" he exclaimed. "Well shall we?"

Chapter 11 The Coming of the Chameleons

"Who is going first," said William as they reached the tree.

"I shall." said H. "Into the future," and he wrapped his scarf around him. The scarf suddenly dangled as though twisting and frolicking in the air. "Wait!" said William, but he had already traveled. The future will be wonderful, so they say but from whose perspective?

So H. found himself in a throng of people. They looked very much like you or me but they communicated through the power of ultimate religious persuasion. Gone were the everyday speech patterns and gestures, the lively relationships: no children played, no lovers loved, no illustrious pageants nor imaginative gatherings. They were chameleons, blending in with the environment; the adventurers of land and sea were reduced to an incessant shuffling! Crosses were the center of their ways- by holding on to these pendants they could have intricate and complex thought patterns. They could live in the dimension and time of their choosing. They existed in these guises, walking, but did so trancelike. They were in fact spending their lives mooching around the world on pilgrimages, searching out the power of holy crosses which were kept in churches to sustain their virtual realities and dimension travel. Each one could be in a medieval joust or in a sun kissed holiday romance or even in deep space exploration, but only in their minds. Mankind had evolved and there was no one to see what had become of them, no characters, nor stop their monstrous reality from existing. Enough of their brain was functional in the real world to get around, seeing through glazed white eyes the obstacles in their way and each was drawn to the specks of light that were the churches.

H., not continually in control, followed the group of pilgrims to their destination. They were heading to what he could only describe as Waltham Abbey. It loomed into view and the participants started to move quicker and more enthusiastically if you could call the shuffling that, and they were soon in view of it. The huge doors were wide open. The people shuffled inside and sat on the pews in such order that was, he thought, the ultimate reverence. His present self fought the will, which made him do so, but his instincts were so highly advanced in comparison that this was easy for him. The difficulty was the flashbacks to where the future self was in the virtual reality-like memories. This infiltrated his thoughts and at moments he was convinced he was laughing and joking with a crowd of virtual people on the coastline art-deco hotel at Walton. He took off the cross and stared about him. Without the illusion of the cross he no longer felt drugged, aware that his surroundings were not the religious experience he thought. There was no light shroud around people, no holy connections. They were in an empty shell of a cathedral, open, overtaken by nature's bounty. The only thing which stood firm was the gold cross which drew the zombies to the alter. Each received the Eucharist by dipping a cup in a disheveled trough of red liquid and held their crosses up to the massive golden cross. To each it was a religious experience that powered their thoughts. To him the energy of mother earth was claiming her victims. He left the place, thinking what purpose life held for the human race. The mind's antipodean spirit was returning back to the flora and fauna from whence it had come. In fact his future self was dragging his thoughts towards the churches. He soon could control this urge and left for the spiral tree. He convinced himself that he would write an account of a Utopian vision in a time traveling book when he got home. The future he concluded was the coming of the chameleons.

Aldous was convinced he would travel to a point in history of his choosing- the context of outlaws. He carved 1738 on the tree and swung himself into the bough. He jumped. Dick and Tom came roaring round the spiral tree just as the metempsychosis was complete. Tom reared his horse but then thundered onward to where Dick was rising over a brow of a hill. Turpin had run into trouble by the road that bisects the Fairlop Oak. The center of Essex festivals, they had stopped a carriage whose business was to root out the outlaws under the 300 feet canopy of the fair lop. It was fortunate that its ample girth had stopped the tirade of musket shot. They were being pursued by the county militia and had covered a mile in only a few minutes but their pursuers were following close in the morning mist. They entered the stubbles but were cut off from escape by a band of men a distance ahead. The breaths of the horses were following dangerously close for comfort. Dick was cut off by a river and thought of hiding in the mill. Aldous had better ideas. There was a cornfield next to the river and two scarecrows stood lapping up the morning sun, not a care in the world. They grabbed the dolls and put on their clothes. They rubbed dirt into their faces and stuffed straw in every conceivable part of their body that was not covered. They then scared the horses and stood limp next to the scarecrow posts.

The militia stormed into the clearing by the river and split up. Some combed the mill while others continued upstream. Two stood where they were and surveyed the scene. Upon noticing the scarecrows they just blinked and upon finding no one at the mill continued upstream where they had found the horses. They obviously thought the fugitives had crossed the river on foot.

Dick was about to prove his real metal. He was a scoundrel. A broad shouldered man was Dick. About five foot nine in his socks, fresh coloured, pockmarked, a light natural wig to cover his head. They waited until there was no sign of the militia and went down to the millpond. Dick however noticed the appearance of a young milkmaid disappearing into a barn. Aldous had come across this form of romance before but Dick was not the kind of man one could say *hold on a minute* to. His present self knew all about his salubrious past. Dick went towards the barn. Aldous stood by the millpond and said: "We are the hollow men, our heads stuffed with straw." Dick's demeanour startled the woman as he stood by the barn door, unbuckling his dishevelled trousers. She giggled.

"I have no other income than scaring crows. Plucking straw from my eyes; hollow men must beauty still. You, my rose, with my heart, my hands on you-which else looks good, as some shade flung from love? Your rights are mine- you have no rights but mine! For I am Dick Turpin, the scarecrow at your service, plucking a dull, river note. This straw is my being. The stiffness of my countenance is your bed. Let me engulf you in earthy passion."

The wooden eaves, couple-coloured like the chestnut mare, beckoned them to the hayloft. He drew currency from the angels to lend an ear from his tender prey. They parted the skies above, limbs and straw entwined. Hayloft riches to impart.

"What dog eat dog? Come let us drink to compliment our escape. We ride together for this fine lady had supplied horses. Let us take our buss to blunder!" Aldous skulked from his musing by the millpond and they took to the saddle heading in the direction of The Kings Head in Chigwell. Dick knew how to get drunk and soon had to be carried up to the inn rooms. He kept going on about something the milkmaid had told him. The millowner's widow had a large chest of gold she kept in the house but which no one knew the whereabouts. This turned his greedy grace into a frenzy. Sure enough the next night Dick and Aldous stood on the hill overlooking the millpond. Dick began in his usual dramatic style.

"The hermit woman beneath this hill has awoken my senses. Her home is in the mill, the lost extremities. Dancing, slowly revolving from the laborers she steals their toiling, who throw shadows as frowns to the Gogmagog hills. Her sorrow their cloaks of silence. Beauty wrapped up in life's cruelty. So strange a will. She awoke my senses. We the giants stop at her sill and like a dream calm her trying. We advance with bounds our heavy bulk covering her neighborhood sounds. Shrouded in clouds, the chills, the stars have produced a vision- says the forest of fools; When your mind's your prison things don't seem so good. But then nobody knows where it goes. When the stars start to shine riches that no one finds. Gold coins are so fine. Her sorrow their cloak of silence. Beauty wrapped up in life's cruelty."

"I suppose you are going to free her from her prison by relinquishing her of her gold?" Said Aldous

"Correct in one", stated Dick and off he strolled in the direction of the mill. Then he remembered her name. His soul froze as he remembered what a newspaper had said on the wall of a pub he frequented. That she was roasted on a spit in order for Dick Turpin to find her chest of gold coins. His heart grew cold and he knew he must stop this perverse act and have it out with him. He trudged down to the mill. The house was dimly lit. Out stumbled Dick with a bag of coins.

"Dog eat dog it was easy", he said. The woman was sitting ashen faced by the fire. "Did you roast her?" Aldous said sternly.

"No" said Dick, "I threatened to but you don't honestly- they both laughed. "She would have made a jolly good roast though." Dick was a scoundrel, a liar and a thief but somehow over the next couple of days Aldous warmed to him. They lived their lives as kings, kings of the forest that is, as Dick never quite knew if a friend was going to betray him. He trusted his friend Tom, and they spent the days wandering and riding round the woods. Dick knew a lot about surviving in the forest and was holed up in a cave in its heart. Not even Tom knew of its whereabouts though. He would travel the length of the Essex Way collecting chestnuts, buying sumptuous meals at taverns and robbing anyone foolish enough to be there after dark. Sometimes though if they had less than a sixpence on them he would give them a crown and send them on their way.

At Fair-Maid-Bottom they robbed a carriage. "Stand and deliver, your money or your life"- Aldous was playing the evil highwayman using his threatening, piecing stare to cajole the gentleman of his generosity, but the man fought back. Dick held the horses and Aldous, caught up in the thrill managed to pass himself off rather well. He got all the money but when he asked for a watch the man opposed him. Aldous did not know what to do but Dick said

"He seems like a good, honest fellow- shall we let him keep his watch?"

"Just do as you will", replied Aldous. The man could, however, not relax until he had promised top pay for it

"Six guineas, we never sell one for more. No questions asked." The man and the two boys were allowed to continue. Aldous was getting quite a taste for the high life of a highwayman. He knew however that his stay was brief. He had a solemn talk with his present self about impending capture and advised him to travel north with no delay at their favorite haunt, the Mole trap. But as Dick said on their parting, the gallows were too good for him. He left Dick and arranged for some of the booty to go with. He traveled to the spiral tree and in an instant was standing in the woods of 1897 with a grand haul of 18th century trinkets. Aldous shook down his clothes.

What had he done by sharing his secret? All Ned knew as he carved his home date on the tree, that life would never be the same again. He wondered of his love, and jumped from the bough. He was in a moonlit, snowy forest clearing. To his horror he found that he was not sitting in his world but had the grim features of an old man!

PART THREE: The Ladder of Time

Chapt. 12 The Ley Towers

For a fuller understanding of what is to follow it is necessary to introduce the warlock of the towers that Ned had disturbed from his forest chamber. That was, is and will be Amaigin.

Amaigin sang a sad song of the futility of life. He was born into a world where intolerance and religion went hand in hand. He was a mischievous lad. His nature was often malicious and he would not see any boundary to his art. His life had sangfroid. He was to all intents and purposes stuck in the body of waiting, and one day found himself carving on the spiral tree. He carved a circle. A zero. He then began to play on the bough, and lifted himself into its branches: he jumped. A noise like a whining of a chimney on a windy day, hollowness that only power invests, enveloped him. He dropped into a throng of black and macabre people. The vampire ring of worship. They were in the center of a burnt earth as if a huge hand had been stoking it for warmth. They stood in a circle and he was one of them. They began to sing

The age of innocence has long since gone
To bite at the nape
Of the tawdry free
Dreaming dreaming in Honilee
For we are part of the never-ending,

Cascade of memory
Lending will to the scape
Shaping will and destiny.

The night on earth may be far too long
To haunt the slain
Ones who never escape
Their mingling in a bawdy room
Convincing others of their doom
As we frighten children witless
Until their mother drunk as fudge
Tucks the well heeled ape
Into a sprig of garlic
And is gone.

Soon an apple was passed to him. He took a bite and a youthful vigor he had long since lost was his. He stepped out of the ring and the change was his undoing. He lost the naivety and only had the blind ambition of youth. Malicious thoughts started to play on the body of waiting. His mind was opening to a whole world of wisdom but he concentrated on its deceit and looking around he wanted. He just wanted. He had the seeds of the ages of the spiral tree and apple of youth. He wanted power. The vampires glimpsed a raven flying overhead and looked up as they headed towards a group of buildings, chatting excitedly and very pleased with themselves, the arrogance of youth restored.

Amaigin sat on his hearthrug, as insatiable as day, the past; rumor and choices, decisions and adventures clearing in his mind. There was a tap, tap, tapping on his mantle door. The raven descended upon the room and changed into the shape of a beautiful girl. He was filled with lust. She stroked her hair and smiled at his barren face. She began to caress him and spoke " You have the world of a youngling at your feet and the wisdom of the ages is in your soul. I have a bargain for you" She went on to explain that the gods needed the apple casket of youth back from the vampires. If he could not help they would turn him to stone.

"But I can do this thing" insisted Amaigin, " Yet the secret of shape-shifting will be given in return." Loki agreed as evening set in. The vampires locked the casket in a strong room and Amaigin opened a grate in the fireplace, room enough for the raven to enter via the chimney. That night the raven entered and upon finding the apples too heavy turned in his mind a hallowed spell to turn it to a nut. Loki lifted it into the still night air with his talons. The vampires, knowing that it was a plan by the gods gave chase, lifting their bat wings into the sky. The raven was growing old and he was slow. However as he reached the battlements of the gods they lit a huge fire. The raven passed through the flames but as the vampires approached they were singed and burnt and fell helpless to the ground dead.

Only Amaigin remained. His youthfulness and his keen eye for treachery were one. He tried to shapeshift but as he said the magic words only a snake was revealed to him. Loki had tricked him. He could only change into the deceitful mind he had become. He went to the spiral tree and carved his home onto the bark. Loki had left him with the mastery of the labyrinthine- that multiple travel was only possible if he stole the innocence of others by gorging on their eyes. Are not fearful passions set up in the soul by a swift concentration of all her energies, her enjoyments, or ideas; as modern chemistry in its caprice, repeats the action of creation by experiment? He had created a monster. To have his will was to perish under the shock of expansion, as the eye trophy killer's plan emerged from the body of time travel.

He hated the religion of his time. Its sickening reliance on sin and virtue. Its humbling belief system. Its bullying tradition of goodness for reward in heaven. Its blind faith in entrenched views whose responsibility was given to God and the devil. He had the sangfroid to treat the void with kid gloves; to respect the magic of his inner and outer worlds. Old ways must be insinuated from the selfish nature of man as all cometh full circle in glory. He must offer the Essex folk that which was theirs, whether they were ready to receive it or not- mathematical reality. He tended towards nature's master plan and use of DNA to abstract from nature the revelation of self-perception through the ways of the b.e.a.s.t. defracted at 45 degrees through the perihelion. The ladder of time; the spiral helix of nature and nurture. Nature by morning climbs in my heart, by noon the sun sustaining by evening we remember the day and as the moon lifts his veil the blue glass wave lifts her hand and strokes the golden shores. Nurtures moment within us will last forever, for we share excitement, enticement, normality here. We will last as undying souls in our paradise created by us, cherished by us. Remembered by us. The ladder of time will be revealed by the thaw of perception.

He constructed a mandate contained within the *labyrinthine*. What you create doth remain in the ether of yesterday's tomorrows. What you hath made doth exist within the pace of the day. Our stay upon this planet may be brief but it is our role in metempsychosis. The soul receives ancestors whose ashes cover our globe with two feet of earth that yields bread to us and flowers. Take it not as religion but mathematical reality. Reclaim the power of nature, the beauty. Man himself will rebuild cities with monsters' teeth, turn night to day with the power of electrons at the speed of light, animate past forests with a lump of coal and fill regions of the soul with perception- without Christianity! As sure as day turneth to night and night to day so the ways of the b.e.a.s.t. will bring revelation through the perception of the perihelion. In the name of rationality, evol insinuated against the void is the ardor of belonging and the spontaneity of the truth. His proclamation was simple. Anguish turns in your soul but perceive through the perihelion and your actions will not be in vain. Not in sorrow but glory. The Christian joke is upon you, what Christ has set down is not the truth. Every human was evol, Christ only a moral teacher of good versus evil who came with a very neat line of nothing in particular.

He prepared to light the torchpaper county with the match of his quarry by building three towers in Essex to rival Stonehenge and Avebury. Replacing piety with instinct. Replacing fear, guilt and obedience with the desire acknowledged by their primitive urges and the tide of nature's loftiness, he built them in Leytonstone and Ingatestone and Walton upon a ley line. Reinforced with the code of nature PHI, 1.618, each was built in dimensions represented by this ratio. The stones positioned thus had the perihelion of the central hall bathed in radiant light each equinox. The crystal prism refracted light at these times with the glory of religious experience. Would love, peace and understanding be so different if labyrinthism, which encouraged expression, self-worth, pride, wisdom and honour, had climbed the ladder of time? If people perceived the supernatural through the ways of the b.e.a.s.t.- surely this would create a moral world unrecognised by permanent divine tradition?

A monstrous phallic, knotted stick with a skull on its tip was Amaigin, and a wry smile crossed his lips. He started across the forest muttering as he went: "I see sense, lost for years, like a circle which never returns. Catching muscles in a net, combining notions like water. Half hold a temple pastiche and chase the pragmatic soul of the plot. Start with a lover by my side, antlers of deer and past pride. For one November in the snow I traverse to the sleeping port." Ned and

Sian finally woke up to their situation but the old man carried on diffidently. "Ardently we walk the boards brooding, for you thought that under lanterns skywards was a birth for two in china-town. A red saffron gown of St. George killing the tolerance is a distraction I would endure but you can't thresh the snow nor touch the belladonna of memories- In the desert we are all blind! Like the currency that brought and upon our hearts daub the desert of the wage; so does your wondrous land my good fortune through history disappear through my hand. As the passage of sand, wasted and wounded, I look for solitude to find reserve- to your room by the roots; same time over, you said leave this place. Strange to pass through as your life gave up the ghost." A raven, a long memoried beast cawed from overhead.

"A raven is controlled by these immortals that are now dead. Once I had a feeling, or should I say she had me, that her covenant; coming from a curious hole, if I can only save its place from my mind map, was that a condition verified maketh the man. Pale you were given to illuminate. Talk I used to listen. But now I can't stop watching, latching onto the smitten expression, I thought I saw your brown eyes turn and once to fire; with her composition flowing beneath crimson sails."

He came upon the lost pond and saw his wizened shape reflected in the moonlight- but there was something shining in his dull sockets tonight. A woman was approaching from the hill and streets of London singing a sweet incantation.

"I am in the London streets on a lonely Saturday night; my feet not fleet, my line not serpentine and my thoughts to you climb. To the spiral tree I went with you, alterwise by moonlight, where I sing, so sweetly sing, a hymn to the wandering Jew, closer to him and further from sin. I'm a London lady, my hems of the Thames, my scarlet ways the gutter my head upon rests. I look up at the Northern star, constantly in the darkness and say where's that at? But this forest edge has lowered me from this canopy, where I am a bird, where my heart does rise. So I wander lonely as a cunt, my head too full to care about my peers, long gone from the just- find my light in a budgerigar, on this wishes edge the only thing I will ask of you is to teach." The old man heard her approaching his cavern and, mumbling madly, hurried on his way:

"I'm too young to die by your dagger! Bright mirror. To find the style of rejuvenation, my extent of creeping is madness- introspective gravity and sublime hysteria. You visit me, you said to have an adventure, but you were all in the future past so I toughen up and face up to reality- We want to label failure so I whirl and fire at the phantoms- Sincere desire reins the moon's face cos I knew how long it would last like wit on board our glistening trail. A spear to lance the wound. I'm only stopping here to halt your passage. On my way stuck in the snow- to draw a confession- that one has to keep a sense of humour. Loneliness like wisdom, which treads a thousand stars on a ride of grace and leaves no print! And leaves no print but a personal fantasy which joins the will, to control above, for salty pride to bring it down. Chances are I will linger in the circle of solitude. Sojourn in a blizzard." His rant subsiding he opened the door of his cavern. He had obviously been affected by the transformation but like any madman, the trouble was to find out how! He closed the hatch behind them.

He had become cold and angry. Winter had come to stay. His selfishness was renown in this age but he was not without followers, such was his wisdom. He had discovered the secret of the Labyrinthine and indeed had written during his travels the books, which enclosed his chamber on Baldwin's Hill. Without the innocence of the witches his life was meaningless, a treatise to vanity, and it had sent him mad. It was in this madman's dream that Ned and Sian found themselves transported. For he was the common link, their common ancestor. As loyal as angels and as seasprung as a sailor, their weblanded feet clung mischievously in the rabbit barren pocked rocks. A rock by any other name Amaigin stared at the young girl. "The rocks are not for throwing today," he said and the books danced the grey sea shanty to cloak their veil of violence upon the land. His disappointment of holding back the tide of history slowly poisoned him. He found to be respected, engulfed in atrocity was to be feared. The raven of peace personified in Jesus was the mercy, which flapped around him still. Like the dusk.

The sorcerer sat quiet and forlorn, a night to enact terrible deeds, with a might in his hands. She stared at the torn, unremitting nature of his face; the same face he saw when looking into the fear of grace. He wished to be purely worn, but the point he will have missed; the dream he shares with countrymen sworn with duty to each harvest kiss, as they lie in the arms of beauty, for the fear of what might be. He recoiled from the daylight with grimace and thunder, for in God's corn of malice and wonder he saw born in the young witches a chance to strike wrong into people he saw as tinder. He sang his lavish song, eyes more hollow than knowledge in power invests. Beseeching lore soaked in lament, he read an apologetic mantra, taunting the power in nature and the land to stop his coven. To campaign against those who held out to be good, he had lacked their conceit of seeing only good and evil. Against forgiveness he had only preached the resolve of metempsychosis. This bore the deceitful ruin at his hest. Only the girl sat attentive, the rest had turned to Christianity. He caressed a snakeform, mustering its depraved intentions to pierce its conquest's resolve as it swung its head from side to side. He was merely a wise conjuror and spoke disappointedly "Where does it go to hide? Is it under the sun, under the earth? Or by the devils side. The age of innocence has far since gone to mock and damn us all from where the people have evil souls and the good are made to crawl. For it sneaks on us from the depths, and grows to immense size, to pounce and drag us down its hole, too far to hear our cries."

He kept vigil at the spiral tree. However he was paranoid that one would come to spite the evil he had created. He hence intended to fell the spiral tree now that he had captured the two travellers of the portal whom he feared would bring his nemesis. He began to prepare for the ceremony, and the ignorance of the girl only added to his power over her. She sighed and he flourished his cape to go outside. They went out to the clearing and on to the spiral tree where a group of young women were gathered, chanting and dancing by a fire, mischief in their souls, evil in their hearts. He touched them provocatively as he felt his libido rise for their deliciously crafted bodies. He started to quieten them and began, like a priest standing over a grave to speak of the treachery of a mind in darkness and the will they needed to replenish, to enter the sewer's earth

The old man then retrieved a pouch from his pocket. As was wished, he poured the contents, the poor dead corpses ashes onto the space by the fire. He then bid the girls to dance upon the corpses ashes. By this he proclaimed the dead would enter into the energy of the gathered throng and be set free. As he did this the girls in a frenzied dance, hooked up their skirts to stamp the ashes into the ground. They did not, however, notice a procession of men drawn towards the fire.

The old man pulled the black cloak into the darkness and was gone. It was the witchfinder general, Matthew Hopkins, a jealous, mean character who had spirited away the love of all things that challenged the entrenched religious views of the time. Some of the party went to the tree and others stood around in mock dismay. The old man however had laid gunpowder around the camp and in the explosive display six witches found escape. However the girl from London, unfamiliar with the territory was rounded up and led away. The first thing Matthew wanted to know was the lair of the warlock.

"Indeed the great face which man thought he saw the devil is alive in this woman. This is good proof that the devil did appear to you in the guise of this man!" There was a contagious silence. "By your silence you then bite on the entrails of goodly men and are the devil incarnate. Is that the truth? The girl denied it vehemently and started to cry to the Lord to forgive her. "Indeed would not all men be haunted as you if the Lord gave them leave. Say you are no more than a puck in this matter, tell us the lair and you will have Gods understanding." His reputation went before him and she was sore afraid. However it was not until boiling water was brought out to cleanse her body that it was that she confessed. Matthew ended the ceremony with a speech praising his good work by the providence of God. Time was catching up with the old man. However madness like the deer the swiftest flew. It seemed like a contagion with which the evil righteous subjected these unfortunate girls to such treatment, rougher justice than any sorcerer ever dealt out.

The general had enticed the warlock out of his cavern to do one last deed. To cut down the spiral tree and not let his secrets fall into the hands of the witchfinder. The old man, looking torn and frayed, thought of the days before the tree, before he had started on his trophy killing. For to travel many times in the labyrinth one needed to steal the innocence of others in the form of their eyes. This secret had warped his mind but made him powerful. As he swung his axe in the early morning mist, a silver dragon; spitting fire arose out of the tree's height. It was Michael's meteor. Michael had pressed his guns on entering the vortex and they now rippled through the trees, ripped into the earth and the swinging arm of the old man!

There was no escape, for although he managed to wind his way back to his cavern, Matthew's host was upon him. They were however terrified, having judged the silver dragon to be the devil's work. Matthew, losing his nerve and the confidence of the party gave the command. As they saw the hatch close he decreed that the warlock be committed to the devils ground. The men piled earth upon the hatch, burying, what they thought forever, the lair of the warlock. The sorcerer who had done great, and evil deeds throughout the vortex of time was finally laid to rest. In the lair he was in crisis. As his existence ebbed away the thought that life had led to this spirit, so without joy nor illusion, pain or pleasure seemed to shed a light on moral dilemma. "Can you find me space inside your bleeding heart" and with that time must have a stop.

Michael's meteor was nearing to the Connaught waters- shell-smooth, rhododendron-colour in the sunrise when he decided to ditch it underneath the water blushing there. He pulled the landing gear handle and swooped at low speed onto a patch of rough ground by the shore. He switched off the engines and let the meteor sink into the mire. He made his way to the spiral tree's forest clearing; it was dawn. In a gully he noticed two children digging frantically with their hands on a mound of earth. He stopped them but one cried

"Amairgin, white knee, is in his cavern under the earth. Please help us to unearth our father". Michael thought for an instance and remembered the evil he had done in the labyrinth.

"Your fathers dead", he replied and then turned to the children. He hung his helmet on a tree and thought. Michael had the knowledge of the labyrinth. He needed to return home to flibbertigibbet. He needed to teach the children-his ancestors, the story between good and evil. For his metempsychosis had revealed to him everything that has and will be and drove him to make amends. He was endowed with the power of change that consumed the land. He caste his mind to the present and travelled labyrinthine!

Chapter 13 The Sky's The Limit

Flibbertigibbet, emotions of sorrow racing faster than wheels in her head was sat by the spiral tree. The tune that was too beautiful to endure, too beautiful to believe played once again. But this time it spoke of pain and loss. She had heard of Michael's death and was distraught. She had the baby in her arms "When we crossed our paths and our hearts what, by chance was lost when we turned away?" she said gently. Their souls moved with the each other's bodies and mysteries unfolded as she took the child in her arms.

"The creations in a lullaby are simple words to keep- the hand that rocks the cradle, wise and caring coven, passed on the starry bone. From a manna comfort; a personality is woven, so lovingly taught a child from wanting stirring the echoes of sleep. The ape in a woman's heart cares for the first-born over the rocks of what ought be the last of the human race like he's a celestial being. The starry bone from my womb torn. Does curiosity never wagered, rekindled in a misspent youth, hide the quality of humankind from youth to age forsooth? Where is my mind, which hides the long wind sane by jumping other people's trains, collecting the success, surety to bide?

Providence comes from carnation of a partnership in love, Oh give me temptation, as pure as the temperance of a dove to light the wonder that tears hide from the thoughts inside. Is the gift of fire the smoke? Only the pride held within. Does the soul collude, to be whispered therein a curious attitude. To spell out mood, in my fruitless coping. My feet scrape like chalk on the steps of the tower. Disposition gloomy and cross, missing the lurch and respecting the loss of faith encased in smoke. I have no faith." Michael dropped out of the tree beside her.

"Have I died? Is this an apparition, a portent of death!" Cried flibbertigibbet.

"No, but a summer's dove, which lightens your mood of love. Let honesty fly through the English sky. Do not stone this dove for its love is ours. Black out the summer sky do, for its beauty is not yours. Hide the strawberries and cream for their taste is not yours." Said Michael

"I long to hear that which lies so near. The honesty whose love lies here. Your hat, your keys, your coat is written in me like a castle's moat protects the maiden dark. To the under-skin, under-heart closer smoothness that is your art, which shimmers and glows. Will this love tear us apart, or keep us together?"

"Let not the stone of life knock it from its flight. Love's honesty kneels, and cries. The sound from its throat; love's first cut healed. Like a lump in the throat. No longer to be feared. Never to be stolen from the kiss of love which is always golden." They kissed.

"Love's first fever was when the sun loved the grass so much that she burned brightly and scorched it and made it wither. Love's second fever is the moon, which quits the sky he does not love. I have had both from the view of my tower"

"Well I am the sun that saves face each morning to bring you happiness" She, who had harboured deep affections for him for so long, was so happy that her heart could burst and they embraced. Power was still at work and played on her distraught sensibilities.

Her's was a world of make believe. She had a fantastic imagination of ogres and dragons, forests and towers, damsels and princes; honed by the realms of medieval fantasy. History to her was but a collective imagination. A great mist folded around her. The stars circled and spun toward her. A dragon appeared out of the starry bone of a constellation and it scooped her from Michael's arms!

The dragon rose into the night sky and soared above a green and forested landscape to an island off the Essex coast, to a tower. There it deposited Flibbertigibbet in the room at the top. She had crawled to safety through the window out from the dragons clutches and it flew away, like silence of departure. But she was alone

The tower had been built around a forest, which had been controlled by four zephyrs. They had met one night. The North wind that was a cold biting wind said, "I can ravage the forest leaves". The south wind that was a warm wind said "I can blow softly and make all the flowers bloom". The east wind said, "I can blow hard and wrench the trees from their roots". The west wind then spoke and said, "I am a swirly, hurly-burly wind and I can make such a noise through the trees that the people will flee". The forest however upon hearing this asked the forest folk to build a wall around the forest and sure enough when the winds howled and blew, the leaves stayed on the trees, no trees fell and the people were not frightened. However the flowers also did not appear. So the people had made a pact with the dragon to steal a damsel and imprison her in the tower to make the flowers grow.

The forest folk surrounded the tower and asked flibbertigibbet a question. We summoned you here to make our flowers grow, by your beauty, but no flowers have grown. Flibbertigibbet was angry and said "Away with you" and they left. They came back morning after morning and asked her the same question. However her resolve was good and every time the answer was the same. "Away with you". Life in the ivory tower was comfortable but bleak. The long nights were lonely and she would pace the floor, bored and forlorn in the daylight that permeated her room. One day when the villagers came she could not stand it any longer and a tear fell from her cheek onto the barren ground. A snowdrop grew. That spring she cried more and more, weeping onto the soft ground beneath and the flowers grew around her ivory tower.

The forest folk were mean and kept her there, or perhaps were frightened but imprisoned her for year after year. The dragon turned up day after day to bring her food and she began to warm to it. Her only friend. He gave her a magic apple each morning, which made her hair grow. She seemed to have an innate fascination for it. It was a deep dark red contrasting with the daffodil yellow star on top, and from side-on it looked like a curled up dormouse for it had one large lump as a head and four smaller lumps in the position of legs. When the apple was finished it transformed from a waxy-red pearl to a carcass that was browning like under the sun's rays. Weeping onto the soft ground she spent every day and night enclosed in her ivory tower, until her hair grew long and grey. Long enough so that the spiralled strands of her hair stretched to the ground.

One day an old knight turned up at the tower. "I have spent my whole life chasing dragons." Said the Knight. "But now I am old and grey and of no use to anyone. Did I grow up too fast?" But when they clinched eyes, though she was old and frail he was inspired. "Nothing I say makes it clear, that you and I have nothing to fear, away from the shy glances, and overdrawn advances, you have waited for me in your ivory tower. You were a princess who belonged to nobody but a burning love. And I'd give up forever to touch you- I will climb the strands of my lover's hair into your heart."

"The flame that I can't conceal from the candle. I went as far as lovers' leap- as far as messing up my sleep under the dying whisper of irony, bereft of the gifts of Byron. Only he sails the briny that comes to me like a tide."

Flibbertigibbet awoke. "Nor England did we know till then!" exclaimed Michael like magic words. For she did not see a frail old man but the majestic, chivalrous stature of Michael's youthful face. She had fainted from the shock of Michael's arrival and she was merely in the arms of her true love in the morning of 1953.

Michael was going to be prepared to time travel. He established his home life and saved money-only in old currency. He awaited the right calendar day in May, wore his flight jacket and proceeded to the spiral tree. He carved 1927 on the bark. He felt pangs of sweet softness as he traveled into the 20's. His purpose was to witness the Spirit of St Louis landing. He walked to the high street and felt a familiar boyhood feel to the place. He stopped off to place a hefty bet on the duration of the flight- 34 hours 30mins and had to stop off at his parents' house to observe from a distance. His family was out for a walk. There he was, swinging in between his parents taking large strides. He looked down on himself and spoke a greeting to his father. He took a bus to Hendon where he bid on, and bought an Avro 504 for £400. He pondered over the controls, put on his flight jacket and took off. It was much like the chipmunks he had trained on, light but maneuverable. He studied the map before take off and navigated a course to Le Bourget Field. His plan was to take off just before the landing and get a magnificent view of the feat. He had been fascinated by the event since he was a child. Today he knew just what to do and tuned in his portable fifties radio to the broadcast, just as he had done as a boy. He could not have lived without seeing this.

Our messenger of peace and goodwill has broken down another barrier of time and space spoke Coolidge, the American president. The silver seabird rose gradually towards the Paris horizon and Michael closed in on him. Bewildered by the frenzy of 100,000 onlookers as Lindbergh stepped out of the plane it was a moment in time. Michael took a picture and then waltzed off in the direction of the Moulin Rouge where he intended top blow his winnings on the heyday of le theatre aux curieux. He fell in love with the charm of the can-can where the dancer's loose jigs hinted at their morals. He returned across the channel to the spiral forest in his Avro. The memory of the Paris nightlife of the 20's was left behind him as he was caught in the vortex to return again to the fifties.

He waited a few years before he traveled to the future to see what aviation had in store. He could not fake it. The world was in a sorry state in 2100. Man had gambled with its future and had paid the price. He brushed shoulders with hideous mutants in the streets and everywhere was on flood warning. There was a close correlation between manufacture and environmental problems. The main environmental consequences of industry were getting out of hand. The use of raw materials and energy in manufacture, and the land-take/pollution in relation to disposal is governed by the law of diminishing returns. There was global imbalance in the developed world. This led to exploitation and a predatory reliance on the third world. Foreign meddling by oversees companies diminished the third world's ability to catch up in wealth. Only seven nations caught up to the west by 2100 (World Bank). The environmental tab of airlines became even more a luxury divide. It led to terrorism. It led to war with the American co-alition. The war machine was getting involved in all major sectors of the world. The planet was in crisis.

If Daedelus were a modern hero his imprisonment of the minotaur would be like the menace of pollution. The effect of pollutants was not fully realized until it was too late. *The silence of the frogs* (New York Times 1992) listed the occurrence of mutation and its genetic relevance to humans. Now mutants were being born to the world at frightening proportion. But this was not the greatest evil. His son's flight too near the sun with waxed feathers would provide excellent analogy to global warming. On September the 11 when all planes were banned in the US the climatic influence was a reduction of 1-2 degrees in surface temperature. Aircraft produce noxious fumes in the lower stratosphere and troposphere – where carbon monoxide, hydrocarbons, nitrogen oxides and methane take longer to break down and have longer term effects. Contrails lead to the build up of cirrus cloud. Nitrous oxide leads to an accumulator effect.

The world of 2100 was in the grips of a rain deluge all around the world. The rise in the watertable coupled with rising sea levels by ice melt at the poles brought a tide of flooding that was catastrophic. Those with the least resources, the least capacity to adapt and were the most vulnerable, were the most affected. The only safe place was in the air. Michael could help in one way with his links to the labyrinthine. Michael was instrumental in working closely with manufacturers to bring about technology Aviators are the springboard to technological growth, and as promoters of this growth they bear a special responsibility for sustainable development. Sustainability was the key to time travel. Sustainability is a state where the demands placed upon the environment by people can be met without reducing the capacity of the environment to provide for future generations. It can also be expressed in the simple terms of a golden rule for the restorative economy: Leave the world better than you found it, take no more than you need, try not to harm life or the environment, make amends if you do. (P. Hawken 1993) It provided an essential resource; time. To Michael, with an overview of the 20th century, development meant to expand or realize the potentialities.

Michaels journey continued in real life after the war. Short duration intervals in specially converted factories kept expectations static: then the answer will always be the same, thought Michael. Consumer demands, conservatism and short-term financial rewards will rule the decisions in engineering, matching performance criteria against sustainability issues. Michael showed the restorative nature of industrial processes. That it is that the true meaning of business is to take responsibility for their product. He showed this responsibility in practise and that life span can be prolonged. He tried to create a value system for the whole life cycle. He rose to the head of engineering at Hawker Siddeley.

LCA and airworthiness techniques paved the way for design impact study. Technology along established research lines led to sustainability targets and newer technologies were not underestimated such as magneto-plasma technology, high mach airbreathing propulsion and hydrogen power. If the vapor problems in the stratosphere can be overcome, all avenues for research have to be guided. Military crossover in the uses of composites and nanotechnology to tailor materials to specific purposes in engines and to reduce weight in structures together with weight saving methods such as bonding instead of riveting were all DFE initiatives he utilized. This is shown no more clearly than in Airbuses concept for the future- the BWB. This used size, aeronautical concepts such as a blended wing, weight saving composites and super efficient high by-pass ratio engines to achieve the future of sustainable aviation. In the skies above Ned and Sian it flew.

He had time to research engineering and was astonished by its results. However he returned with an analogy of time travel: sustaining the past by your actions was to sustain the future in your present. He vowed to change the world of aviation for a greener future. He established himself as a visionary engineer with the vision of the future state of play behind him but time-travel had taken a toll on his health.

He waited until he had finished the foundations of his dream and had risen in management. He decided to again take precautions. He had many flight hours in a spitfire of the 60's. He took the identity of a downed fighter pilot and sifted religiously through the records to get his story and uniform correct. Cloaked without a sound he carved the date of the start of the battle of Britain on the bark and jumped like he was floating down on a parachute into 1940.

He would be unleashed in a wartime spitfire today and as he saw the elliptical shape of the spitfires in the sky above the airfield of Waterbeach, a strange heady mix of elation and fear gripped him, calmed by his maturity. He was welcomed as a pilot of rare ability and caliber. He insisted upon taking the place of a raw recruit who was destined to die in the affray. He forewarned the squadron of the nature of the German onslaught and why the only thing was to get at 'em boys.

They were sufficiently prepared to be the first squadron to engage the bombers, foiled quickly by the Duxford wing, led by the legendary Douglas Bader. The sortie followed an astern formation, which Michael had learnt at the helm of the twin nacelled meteor. A big wing of six squadrons dived in simultaneously from all directions and the Germans were soon frantically keeping to formation and hiding amongst the ME109's that

136

were in disarray at the surprised onslaught of the big wing.

"Bandits now at ten o'clock" urged Michael as he saw three ME109s climbing fast to get enough height to strike and attacked them before they had a chance. He engaged a German as it passed through the astern formation, banked and followed up with a tirade of gunfire. He stuck on its tail and unleashed his guns at its rear. He was endeavoring to line up his guns once again but held his fire as he saw the hood open and the pilot plunge out, the plane plummeting in the churning air. He swept into a ball of smoke- for a moment he thought he was under fire. The planes then concentrated upon the bombers and Michael dispatched a Dernier with a burst of gunfire. It exploded with such force that the neighbor banked and bucketed to the ground. The bombers had reached the flack of London and the Me109s had all but given up the ghost. One was careering towards the forest canopy and Michael gave chase. His guns ripped into the fuselage but the pilot was aiming for the vortex opened by the spiral tree. Michael followed him in. The power of the land had consumed them and the crippled German landed in 1963. When Michael ripped open the cockpit he was unconscious but proved to be a respectable fellow. Michael took him to the spiral tree and sent him on his way, having first reconnoitered his ME109. The museum had its two prize exhibits.

The more theory defined physical laws and the more practice stretched the boundaries, the more those boundaries became blurred. It is only right and proper that the task of defining the boundaries should come from blurring time's laws themselves. Unlike Amaigin Michael chose to sustain the future by travelling into the past. It gave him the strength to do what was impossible, the sense to not attempt the impossible and the wisdom to know the difference.

Chapter 14 Embers of an Elizabethan Hunt

Michael had lived for his business with Peter. It was a museum called Aces High containing the relics he had recaloitered from his labyrinthine travels. One evening the two friends were at the Royal Forest pub when they noticed a large orange moon over the Queen Elizabeth hunting lodge. Peter mentioned the strange sensation he had of feeling pomp and magnificence from the carpark to the verge.

"I've always wanted to see what it was like at a hunt." He said

"Do you want to find out?" Replied Michael. Michael went on to tell him of the significance of the spiral tree. Not one to lie, Peter was amazed by this and they arranged to sleep on the idea and met by the forest the following afternoon.

Peter carved 1588 onto the tree and jumped from the bough. He found himself leashed to a dog, a massive grey-muzzled dog. The dog led him to where he could faintly make out the sound of the beaters. The path to Buckhurst hill was awash with finely clad hunters and hangers on. He followed the procession, and requisitioned a horse to join the affray. The queen sat, side-saddle on a great chestnut mare. Of course like the Christian mythology that says that you already know everything there is to know it's just that you have to reach that knowledge though accepting the plateau of experience, and deliverance; she could unlock emotions. The labyrinth is self-discovery, so that he could see the wondrous nature of ecology, open to the charms of life again by her majestic form. Her courtiers beckoned to him and he joined her.

"Will someone please tell me what is going on!" She commanded abruptly

"Well," said Peter "I think you will find that the deer has gone to ground somewhere in the bushes." Just as he said that a five-point buck rushed from the bushes, thick pelted and monstrously snorting, ahead of them. Peter drew his bow and took aim. The beast dropped where it stood.

"Marvelous. We have dinner tonight. You will join me of course?" They proceeded to the lodge but the queen dismissed her entourage and continued with a small band of loyal courtiers. She moaned about the hangers on at the lodge and summarily dismissed them telling a courtier to arrange a *small* feast of venison for her guests.

"For the greater glory of England, a vast and secure vestry. At its heart its home, politics, philosophy, its army, unveils the story of history. Vikings from dark ages spread their warrior life dependant upon raiding. Wedded to the sea even in dread. An unholy, macabre reigning, individuals against the coastline were the fragility of English constancy. And they ravaged the land to charcoal. To vanish from history's recall. Shaped by ancient embers. Transient people tolerance stood, demonised by modern plunder, with golden bow pushed westward, the Spanish with splendour and wonder, impressed on us like the sword they used to win territory. Side by side like mountains they grew rich from empire shaped from ancient embers. We must show no fear yet be insecure enough to see the truth: we need to stay in a state of suspended animation, like a work of art" She spoke to him as though they were anything but acquaintances of a hunt but the wine flowed and the food was sumptuous so that he decided to talk in the manner to which he hardly dared:

"A woman's trust is strange. Love is strange; I heard this once, the new things from the old times known. The innocence whose frailty grown into the mystic, worldly wise and in the night we fled, we understood the tenor of a young man's guise to be a collector of all that's new- a love I beheld when I met you. But was it new or past familiarity been: in the keenness of youth, or a strain for melody long since seen. This delicate truth- and in the night we fled, we understood- of woman who instantly recognises sense, which breaks the mould and heals the henceforth future torn of momentums brow; the marmalade trout of the here and now. When will the icicle melt, the emotions that flood in spring's flaming wound, from my grave expression to your glorious bud. For in the night we fled, we understood- a queen's resolve for her country, her mignons, the harmony I decree is our very essence, the manna born. From each new emotion. The part of your heart you with us leave and lay it upon your new greensleeves."

"I refuse to make windows into men's souls ... there is only one Jesus Christ and all the rest is a dispute over trifles".

"- those moments where you were not clear, not focused rather a scrunched up piece of impudent feeling and hurt pride." He replied, but it was too much for the well-guarded queen, who put her finger to her lip. The queen was made vulnerable by the political climate of Spanish ascendancy and she soon made her excuses. She went to the upper private chambers. All was dark and the owls hooted as the deer ran from their pens into the midnight air. The embers of the fire were dulling and there was movement among the guests whom were in corners discussing things of very little importance. Peter took his leave. He stared out at the orange moon and at the white Tudor building. Te voir a illuminaire mon coeur. The moon drips ivory blossom.

Lust for power was as a demon seed blowing upon the wind ever attracted to that which was pure and delineated by her form. Only in his mind did the hands movements caress the firm ripe joints of the victim, cajoled and harried the prey until it was trusting and its loyalty faded into a patch full of secrets, to be welcomed but not, understood. As he thought so, something caught his eye. Movement at the upper window. The queen, dressed in a long flowing white nightgown dropped in a flurry a white handkerchief from the window then was gone. His cottage was along the forested way of Epping and Hatfield forests where he had first spied the queen playing with the Earl of Essex as children. Fickleness was manifested in the symbol of love she lavished upon this relationship. Like the wind proceeded the rain he decided to stay on at the Kings head and follow her to London.

It dawned on the queen as she traveled that this was to be like the journey when she was summoned to the tower; that it was to test her resolve as a woman and as a leader. She felt comforted by the arrival of Sir Walter Raleigh. He was born from the river, born of mud and filth. The dirty city beckoned to him and when the dirty city had quenched his passions and given him a bone all of his own, he desired the seas. Foe were born of the river, but were dead at his hands, shrink wrapped in their own skin, in their own graves before he had even left these shores to seek fortune and deception. One wave-tossed day he had sailed one hundred leagues or more, and the men outside and rats, which scratched, were calling to the saints to drive a dagger in his eye. He thrashed the ringleader and carved a skull and dagger into his chest. Such was the resolve of this man. Peter kept his distance and the queen through the whole journey kept stern contact with her advisors. He was yesterday's tender prey.

He listened to her speech to her troops on the Sussex downs, and was impressed by her attitude: *Let tyrants fear; I have always so behaved myself that, under God, I have placed my chiefest strength and safeguard in the loyal hearts and good will of my subjects. And therefore I am come amongst you at this time, not as for my recreation or sport, but being resolved, in the midst and heat of the battle, to live or die amongst you all; to lay down, for my God, and for my kingdom, and for my people, my honour and my blood, even the dust. I know I have but the body of a weak and feeble woman; but I have the heart of a king, and of a king of England, too.*

Chapter 15 A Faerie Love

Ned had been witness to a faerie love in his youth. He had met Sian on the beach and as children had played in the Martello tower, the forest and the sand. All that Ned had left before was his sense of humour. He had been nothing but a gala man. The decisions, which had been made for him, had extraneously changed his life for the worst. But now he had Michael. The web he was to spin became their childhood faerie beds. Flibbertigibbet had told them stories of adventures so real that they fuelled their imagination and left an indelible mark on their minds. Their favourite was the swan that thought it was a bear. There was a crack and a split and the egg revealed its occupant. There among the reeds was a cygnet. Grey and huddled it began to waddle towards a strange bunch of brown reeds. It nestled there and fell asleep. As if there was an earthquake the reeds started to move and a funny brown face looked down upon the cygnet. "Daddy" said the cygnet. "Growl" went mound of brown reeds, and the most astonishing half growl was returned to the bear. The bear, thinking nothing of it, headed towards the forest. The little swan followed. Over the mossy fields, boulders and tree-lined bogs went the two figures. The bear eventually looked round and saw the little swan following it. "Growl" went the bear and sure enough the cygnet growled back, enjoying the game of follow my leader. The bear, thinking it was silly for a swan to think he was a bear, gave a hearty laugh and rubbed himself on a tree. The cygnet followed suit. All through the summer the bear likened to the swan and went about teaching it all the bear things to do. He was especially capable at fishing and they ate well. One day while fishing in the late evening, a flock of swans approached, chattering excitedly. The swan growled and the astonished swans took flight. All but one, a snow-white female. But the swan turned his back on her. The swan that thought it was a bear preferred being a bear.

This was Ned's past life. Previously both had lived a full life, apart, but one thing remained; the further did not take away from the nearer for there had been something lacking in their thrill-seeking thoughts that were wed from experience and the dull tree lined streets of their youth. Scholarship is the enemy of romance and money has and never will bring people together but these were the simple things that had driven them apart. He had few illusions for Michael taught him well and arranged for them to grow up together by not moving from their village in Chigwell Row. Sian he knew was a true friend before anything could draw them apart. Michael then employed her as interior designer at a museum he owned with Peter and Ned.

Destiny folded up like the waves over a boat of sand. Their relationship was crisp and natural like the apple. They always made each other feel brilliant, even after disappointment. Well I know that is a bit depressing but quite true. They had serious moments when they needed them-they didn't rely upon the jack-the-lad mentality. They could address issues neither of them felt comfortable with ease. They were light, wise and approachable. They appreciated the finer things in life. They were both centred and did not pander to the qualities of excess- unless they wanted to. He felt like a free spirit when he was with her and soared to new heights just thinking of her. They were both insane but had a firm hand on reality. She was dangerously sexy when she got serious. She was dangerously sexy when she had clothes on. In fact she was dangerously sexy. She could make his lowest resolution spark into fruition. He was encouraging and as interesting as she was beguiling. They wrote extremely valuable poetry and they were honest as the wings by which they fanned desire- so as not to ever let it burn out. She was a marvellously inspired and fantastical writer of music. With her music comes ideals and beauty the like of which is only dreamt about. He had a scientific mind and a balance to which the coolest surfer boy would be proud. They were amazing in their idealism and grounded in their optimism. She did not mind if he got slightly obsessed. They were mysterious and strange.

Each moment passed surpassing the next and they would play games out of the moist regions of their mind, talk, and create small ceremonies of the mundane aspects of their lives. He was so much in love that when they drank a glass of wine she had to peel him off the ceiling. They could write letters of love and ideas to each other. Her opinions were so correct. Her ideas sent him up in the clouds searching for reasons. They were both happy, but mordantly sanguine. She gets embarrassed when he compliments her. She always hit the mark. She has the ability to be joyously honest and never form an opinion which is hearsay nor malicious. They were fair to the end but darkly sardonic and though wistful had an amazing intelligence which cuts through nonsense like a cat through the sinew of prey. She had a wicked sense of humor and was as fun as the blow up furniture on swimming pools is tacky. They held little pretension but it was well founded when they did. She turned a heavenly day into delicious sin and every day into heaven. Intimacy was her desire and to be intimate with her was to stand on the shoulders of giants. To be lovers was exquisite, her friend a dream. Her ways of the heart; her belonging, her evil, her ardor, her spontaneity and her truth were all-intact and guided his emotions running beneath his skin. Surpassed was his romantic self-destruction of his other life in an ivory tower. Surpassed was his depression of living for stokes to enhance his mood.

So their relationship progressed and the two sang a sentimental song of excitement, enticement and normality. As the14th moon lifted his veil Ned finally managed to propose. It was Valentines Day and he wrote her a poem in a card:

My everything, my nightly Honilee, my summer's kiss

A faerie love did bless
The future sealed with a kiss
Its secret sap arising
As a tree which blooms each spring
And blossoms for the chastened, fairer sun to play
upon
To bare the toils
Its boughs, its leaves, its glory
Its fronds beseech
A happy home beneath
A sky so full of joy that unicorns do fly
Upon a windswept apogee
Of earths great livery
And spread its meteor plumes
That reach into your secret night
To forge the finest, shining, glittering ring
Shared for eternity
All our wonders everlasting
All our happiness enchanting

"I do love nothing in the world as well as you, is that not strange?" She replied.

Chapter 16 Time's Laughing Stock

Ned stood on the same day in 1979 as when he travelled Labyrinthine. This time though he had been advised by his father to throw the book into the spiral tree. This was a father's solemn advice and he did so. His reasoning was that the tapestry of life was ruled by innocence and madness and through innocence came abandon and through madness understanding. A paradox. Secrets are often best kept hidden. Great danger awaited Ned in the past.

The book fluttered and scattered into the trees ample bough. He saw his thoughts turn to the lost souls of heaven who walk on the ground and within a labyrinth of ancient memory his mind stretched and swung from the lives of his ancestors. Time played upon him. A mist closed around him as he travelled labyrinthine. There was a rush of wind. Trapped in the labyrinth he saw, or rather lived a huge schism of other worlds; mysterious, wonderful, dreadful, and sinful which soothed like angels and cut like barbed wire and maggots. Eventually it calmed down to a scene of hill and vale. Many different coloured marble stones lay strewn about and there was a raven on the spiral tree with the feeling one gets when the first snow falls.

The raven cawed incessantly and doves flocked into a perfect circle, brighter and brighter until the aura became a sphere and tunnelled forward. The raven cawed a final time then exploded into a rainbow that lead straight into a tunnel. The rainbow became a thin stream of life's decisions. He knew all the colours they were; gold belonging of memories, black evil of chill waters, blue the ardour of the sky above, red spontaneity of cabernet sauvignon and green the truth of futures not written in stone. Life's decisions seemed open to him and he held destiny in his hand like an apple.

The rainbow path hummed slightly and everywhere was surrounded by a tranquil pure white light. From the distance a lady appeared walking down the rainbow path. Lifting up her dress she spoke; "Come, come child at ease, I am so powerful but even I let some things slip. So many words and so many friends but I too have come from the after-void. Void was before, now and future- It is above and beyond. My minions have been so loyal but the void is strong and finds its way into the spirit © Oliver Dachinger. Earth is such a turbulent place that the void balances the forces of nature. But I have made a mistake. The void has triumphed. *It has been encoded in their genetic make up, too virulent to control. I did not want this. I told the angels to encrypt Gods plaque in their genes but Lucifer under influence of the void tampered the instruction into void plague* © Oliver Dachinger. Mankind is trapped by its own volition" She calmed herself. "The ways of the b.e.a.s.t. is the challenge."

They were riding down the rainbow on a sledge pulled by a half dog, half reindeer like creature. They realised the source of the rainbow at a prismatic perihelion, which refracted dimensions to him like he was opening the doors of perception in a labyrinth. It interfaced with your reality and sent your subconscious potential, with the responsibility of your conscious, through dimensional discovery. As they looked into mystery it was a childhood scene, the hustled adulation of a crowd, the peace of a country village, the dismay of missing someone; but overriding it all, a feeling of fulfilment in a moment of truth until they were floating on hope and fear. He felt at one with his surroundings but part of it and emanating from herself and the feeling, closer than fiction, was the mystery of cherished moments exploding from pinnacles of light.

"Simultaneous but individual, the five ways of the b.e.a.s.t. will guide you to perceive the mist rising on a whole nether world of sparking and longing illusion. Time affects the labyrinth's shape through this perihelion, a prismatic sunflower of sunrise projecting belonging, evil, ardour, spontaneity and truth." In the past his ivory tower of innocence and madness of the void had taken over destiny; destiny where thought was the slave of life and life was time's fool. The spectre of time, which made one brave the slave of disorder had made a crucial mistake, compounded by mankind.

Ned was handed a ticket by the strange spectre before she turned into a raven and flew away. He passed a couple on the way to the doors of the tower. He felt for an instance he recognised her. He barged his way through he malingerers of the void who were trying to blag their way in with false tickets and his stub was handed back to him.

Down a corridor of the passing years with longing as gravity, and ideas as direction and emotion as motion, was a room. It was at once huge like Westminster hall with drawing boards by which you pieced together the past- drawn by the future. A mirror illuminated mysterious staircases winding downwards and upwards full of familiarity been and he watched himself as his ancestors moulded into his face. His face was transfigured in the impossible paradox that reality is totally; indefinitely present in all particulars. It was a perspective of belonging. If in belonging she would take to him and this was seen as good.

Ned entered through the curtains to a backstage area. There grotesque but sexy gypsies with make-up of the most extreme void pranced and held their poses of sexual allure. Temptation presented by the void and flaunted for what purpose, only perversion knew. A whip cracked and for a moment he wondered if it was in his power to wield the whip. They had exceeded expectations made of them by using and abusing money and power. And as a consequence life had diminuted into a tirade of self-abuse and possessions. It was a measure of perception that made them the mechanism of the material void. He had made his decision by not following the fantasy of easy sex which pervades every monkey coming, pushing them to the floor and joining the monkey orgy. He had not succumbed to evil encased in wrath to contaminate the bed, which sealed men's fate. He climbed the stairs and opened a door at the top.

Ned shook down his clothes. He was dressed in black, a chain male doublet and trousers with circular belt buckle of ancient runes on it. Time's bell tolled, by morning showed, the night concealed the ramparts of the tower below him, hewn from the rock face itself, where the opulence of the ruling elite was ensured. He stepped away from himself...the restorative nature of life itself was revealed to him... the secret... in the tower of memories, the talisman of fortune and coincidence, enlightenment of expression shared with others... the pointless journey to death... in some overlooked ancient rune, in some overlooked intellectual sensibility, the ecological instinct of the code of PHI... in the ladder of time-in love itself perhaps?

Or so it seemed for the tower was locked in the mists, which surrounded him like instincts, mixed with a heady concoction of power and wisdom. The realization dawned on him as the sun's majesty broke through. That the void was just an empty edge without the ways of the b.e.a.s.t. perceived through the perihelion. Without it the code of chance would very nearly turn one mad. Dignity towered above the pagan landscape as a raven fluttered on the flag for it was no place for the meek. Its river ran red all over the Essex to quench the golden corn of the harvest. St George had not killed the dragon and St. Patrick not banished the snakes so that the animal kingdom had merged into the human world and the men, took on the form and the manner of beasts. Ned's mask was black like the raven.

It clung to the coast where the sea rose and fell. After it had ravaged the coast many came and went as it had done. Fire was heard in the heartland. He beat down heavily upon ignorance's tattered standard. Its frenzied, pinpoint accurate attacks broke the screams of the dying and taunts of the bloodied hoards. It is strange to me that beauty is often slain in the night as a raven fluttered on the flag; the emblem of dignity through lone mercy we find out things that we do not through experience of consoled abandonment just as in the dark ages. It is the measure of a man to adjust and then purpose flux to cause the raven of mercy to jump through the disc of the inferno. The raven visibly healed those in battle worn- and its response to faithful men was to leap the ravine spread like faith to the eye of mercy.

As he stood on the brink he began to think of his belonging to the animal kingdom. His sinews flexed and the reality relented until wings gifted his senses with truth and spontaneity. The empty edge of the void shattered his thin veil of illusion. But he knew what he must do. The drop from the tower would not be to fall but to soar. He mustered himself and plunged toward the sea at the foundations of the tower. The walls checked his progress as he dived, dived into the black waters of evil. He felt a life force stir and slow his acceleration, parrying the rushing winds with his wings. He plunged into the icy waters. He was drawn to the pools and pikes plunged left and right of him but they seemed as shadows and left no mark on him. He pulled himself out of the water and walked upright and forthright to the gates. He pulled on them, stepped back and mustered his ardor. They turned to a curtain of fluid dreams and he walked through the thick iron bars. Love only made one believe in what won't happen and proved nothing to be true. The truth of innocence lies in disbelief. This is the paradox of time grafted from the heart of the beast.

He was transported to the beginning of the journey and was outside in the rain of the street with the apple in his hand; then the familiar couple passed him. What do you get for being in love anyway? Quoth the void. But Ned was animated and spontaneity held out the apple. Sian, for some reason, trusted him and took a bite and they walked through the tower portal. They were again holding hands, walking in a sunlit village, beautiful old gardens full of grass and flowers and trees. All clocks were stopped and told only dandelion time. A country road stretched into the distance lined by walnut trees. This was the open future, too impossible to believe, too beautiful to endure played on the strands of his lover's hair. Nature spoke to him like a code. A code which enlightened him to realize that the truth of life was that we always knew what to do- if only one perceives that life is discovery not the accumulation of knowledge per se. The truth lay all around him, scattered like the flowers of a meadow at his feet, and the love she bore was innocent. I loved innocence more than health or beauty, preferred her to the light since her radiance never sleeps. In her company and at her hands riches are not to be numbered. The ladder which was lost in the snow has been found. The ivory tower on that day breached. Innocence had consumed madness.

Printed in the United Kingdom
by Lightning Source UK Ltd.
118648UK00001B/79-117